Principles and Practice of
Psychiatric Nursing

Principles and Practice of
Psychiatric Nursing

TP Prema BSc (N) MS (USA) PhD
Professor and Principal
Sanjay Gandhi College of Nursing
SGAH & RI (Sanjay Gandhi Accident Hospital and
Research Institute), Jaya Nagar East
Bangalore

KF Graicy BSc (N) MSc(N)
Nursing Tutor
NIMHANS, Bangalore

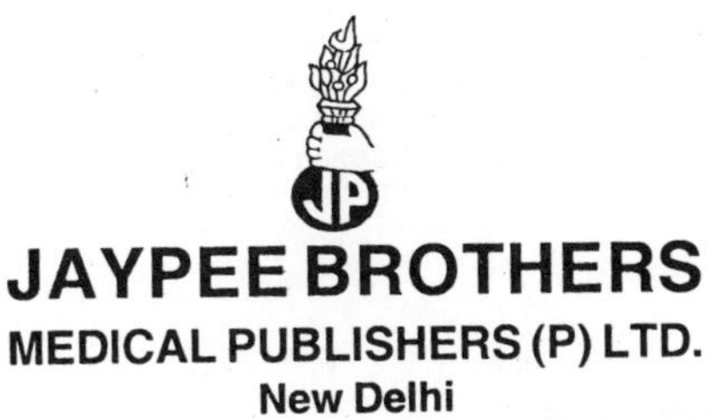

JAYPEE BROTHERS
MEDICAL PUBLISHERS (P) LTD.
New Delhi

Published by

Jitendar P Vij
Jaypee Brothers Medical Publishers (P) Ltd
EMCA House, 23/23B Ansari Road, Daryaganj
New Delhi 110 002, India
Phones: +91-11-23272143, +91-11-23272703, +91-11-23282021, +91-11-23245672
Fax: +91-11-23276490, +91-11-23245683
e-mail: jaypee@jaypeebrothers.com
Visit our website: www.jaypeebrothers.com

Branches

- 2/B, Akruti Society, Jodhpur Gam Road Satellite, **Ahmedabad** 380 015
  Phone: +91-079-30988717 e-mail: jpamdvd@rediffmail.com
- 202 Batavia Chambers, 8 Kumara Krupa Road, Kumara Park East
  Bangalore 560 001 Phones: +91-80-22285971, +91-80-22382956,
  +91-80-30614073, Tele Fax: +91-80-22281761 e-mail: jaypeemedpub@eth.net
- 282 IIIrd Floor, Khaleel Shirazi Estate, Fountain Plaza, Pantheon Road
  Chennai 600 008 Phones: +91-44-28262665, +91-44-28269897
  Fax: +91-44-28262331 e-mail: jpchen@eth.net
- 4-2-1067/1-3, Ist Floor, Balaji Building, Ramkote, Cross Road
  Hyderabad 500 095 Phones: +91-40-55610020, +91-40-24758498
  Fax: +91-40-24758499 e-mail: jpmedpub@rediffmail.com
- 1A Indian Mirror Street, Wellington Square **Kolkata** 700 013
  Phones: +91-33-22456075, +91-33-22451926 Fax: +91-33-22456075
  e-mail: jpbcal@cal.vsnl.net.in
- 106 Amit Industrial Estate, 61 Dr SS Rao Road, Near MGM Hospital, Parel,
  Mumbai 400 012 Phones: +91-22-24124863, +91-22-24104532,
  +91-22-30926896 Fax: +91-22-24160828 e-mail: jpmedpub@bom7.vsnl.net.in
- "KAMALPUSHPA" 38, Reshimbag, Opp. Mohota Science College, Umred Road
  Nagpur 440 009, Phone: +91-0712-3945220, +91-712-2704275
  e-mail: jpmednagpur@rediffmail.com

Principles and Practice of Psychiatric Nursing

This book has been published in good faith that the material provided by authors is original. Every effort is made to ensure accuracy of material, but the publisher, printer and authors will not be held responsible for any inadvertent error(s). In case of any dispute, all legal matters are to be settled under Delhi jurisdiction only.

First Edition: **2006**

ISBN 81-8061-614-2

Typeset at JPBMP typesetting unit
Printed at Sanat Printer, Kundli.

PREFACE

The authors of the book *Neurological and Neurosurgical Nursing* published in 2002 have decided to have another one titled *Principles and Practice of Psychiatric Nursing*. in 2006. Everyone in the medical and paramedical field, knows about the clear relationship between neuro-science and behavioral science. Since the authors work in NIMHANS, the premier institute, which stands as the model for this relationship, they have the right to compile few chapters on psychiatric nursing. Their knowledge in theory and experience in clinicals helped them complete this work. Great leaders in nursing in India and abroad have given their valuable views about Psychiatric Nursing in different texts. But here the authors give their views, based on the previous texts which are prevailing in the market for many years, and their experience in different areas of psychiatry. Their experiences include a acute psychiatry, chronic psychiatry, child and adolescent psychiatry, community psychiatry, psychiatric rehabilitation, etc.

This book is divided into 29 chapters and these 29 chapters are grouped into 6 units.

Ist unit briefs review of psychiatric nursing, concepts of mental health, mental illness, principles of psychiatric nursing and all aspects of history taking in psychiatric nursing.

Second unit consists of 5 chapters and describes the causes, classification and few modalities used to modify the maladaptive behaviors, different techniques of communication and therapeutic interpersonal relationship.

Third unit discusses about the nurses' responsibilities while nursing the individuals with behavioral problems.

It includes psychotic conditions, neurotic conditions, mental retardation, organic mental disorders and childhood disorders.

Fourth unit has 4 chapters. It includes the admission-discharge procedures, legal responsibilities of nurses, the difference between Indian Lunacy Act (1912) and Mental Health Act (1987). It also gives the importance of records and reports in psychiatric nursing.

Fifth unit describes the nurses' responsibilities in emergency care of individuals with maladaptive behaviors and nurses' role in rehabilitating them. Pharmacotherapy has an important role in the field of psychiatry. This unit talks about the nurses' role while nursing these individuals when they are on medications. The nurses should have knowledge about the names of drugs, dosages, routes of administration, indications and contraindications, etc. They also should have knowledge about the side effects and their immediate treatment. So these chapters give the information about the drugs used for these patients.

Sixth and last unit gives the common nursing problems found in psychiatric wards and their interventions. This era is the era of community nursing. The psychiatry also heading towards the community to get the resources available to prevent, treat and rehabilitate the psychiatric patients.

A glossary is enclosed at the end of this book.

We acknowledge everyone who helped and encouraged us directly or indirectly to complete this work. Above all we are grateful to His providence for inspiration and guidance throughout this work.

TP Prema
KF Graicy

CONTENTS

CHAPTER 1

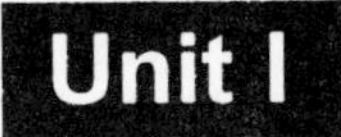

Review of Psychiatric Nursing

INTRODUCTION

Nursing or caring the sick is an art in itself. It is a need-based art, which inherited not only to human beings but to animal kingdom also. Often we see an animal in need is helped or nursed by another, it is fed, carried and even protected.

In early human history family members, servants, friends, neighbours and some religious groups carried out the nursing or caring the sick. Later these activities were carried out by women for their livelihood, till the middle of 18th century. Around this time the scientific knowledge was gradually added to this nursing art.

Florence Nightingale, who is known as the mother of modern nursing formulated the scientific reasons for the nursing work. She discussed about disease conditions, causes, causative organisms, route of entry of microorganisms into human body and also the importance of environmental hygiene in the maintenance of health. She also told that nurse could cause infections to the patients if she does not practice aseptic techniques while she does wound dressing and other procedures. The nursing could be defined as an art and science, when the original art is combined with scientific knowledge and reasoning.

At different periods of history, different scholars viewed nursing, in their own words. Some of them are mentioned here. The unique function of nurse is to assist the individuals, those activities contributing health or its recovery or to a peaceful death, that she would perform unaided if she had strength, will or knowledge to help the patient to gain independence as rapidly as possible (Henderson, 1966) Watson states Nursing is a service of caring (1979). The type of nurse required today is one who possesses an all-around personality, the required general education and prescribed professional education. She should have a desired degree of maturity with possibility of development to enable her to work effectively with in the community. She should be competent enough to share professional responsibility as a member of health team in treating the sick (Government of India, 1989).

The present day nurse is an encounter with a client and his/her family, wherein the nurse observes, supports, communicates, ministers and teaches. She also contributes to the maintenance of optimum health and provides care during illness until the client is able to assume responsibility for the fulfillment of his own basic needs. In other words the nurse has the responsibility not only in the hospital, but also to take care of the client to get rehabilitated to his maximum functional ability within the limits of the prognosis of disease he is affected.

Because of the different views of different leaders, in the last two centuries nursing is gone through several changes. These changes happened due to changes in nursing curriculum, medical practices, economy of developed and developing countries, in the political scenario and the facilities available to treat and rehabilitate the patients. In the nursing education and practice, important points to remember are the courses available in different specialities like diplomas in critical care nursing, operation theater nursing, oncology nursing, neuroscience nursing. Nursing for psychiatric patients also turned into speciality nursing for the last few decades. Psychiatric nursing underwent many evolutions before it turned into a speciality nursing. Few important leaders and their contributions to psychiatric nursing are discussed below.

Linda Richard who graduated in 1873 from New England Hospital developed better nursing care in psychiatric hospitals and organized educational program in the state Mental Hospital of England. For this reason she is known as the first psychiatric nurse. During her times in Malian Hospital (WAVERLY), the first school of nursing opened to prepare nurses to care for mentally ill. The importance of Linda's program was, it prepared the nurses to assess both physical and emotional needs of patients.

In 1913, John Hopkins was the first school of nursing to include a fully developed course curriculum to prepare the psychiatric nurse.

Along with the prescribed curriculum nursing leaders started defining the psychiatric nursing and listed down some unique functions of psychiatric nurse, Stockwell (1985) defined psychiatric nursing as a complex, skilled planned activity that aim the teamwork and co-operation at restoring full health functioning of mentally ill individuals, minimizing the defect or disabilities arising form gross illness or institutional care, protecting the individual from harming himself or others.

Peplau (1952) in her book "Interpersonal Relation in Nursing" described the skills, activities and role of the psychiatric nurse. She believed the four phases of interpersonal relationship (orientation, identification, exploration and resolution) should be practiced by the psychiatric nurse, while taking care of her clients. In 1953, National League for Nurses (America)' published a study of desirable functions and qualifications for psychiatric nurse.

This report identified the following desirable functions for psychiatric nurse:

1. Collecting the significant data relating to identification of problem in observing the behavior of patient and recording them.
2. Making inferences and judgment based on these data and leading to action, i.e. interpreting the behavior of the patient.
3. Acting and intervening on the basis of inferences.
4. Evaluating the entire process in terms of whether problems are solved.

By 1960, the services of the psychiatric nurse is extended to different areas other than inpatient settings. The extended areas are outpatient department, partial hospitalization, community services, emergency services, consultations and even teaching. She is included in the health team of doctors, clinical psychologist, psychiatric social workers, occupational therapist, etc. If one looks at the evolution in psychiatry one can equate the changes happened in the psychiatric nursing also especially in 20th century.

Till Philippe Pinal broke the chains of psychiatric patients in 1792, they were given only institutional care in lunatic asylums. During that period nurse also was assigned to do the minimum basic needs for these individuals and the last rites after death.

Fraud the Father of Psychology established that the fixation theory at different stages (Oral, anal, phallic) in childhood, make the individual to behave abnormally sometimes or the other in their lifetime. He practiced behavioral therapies to modify the abnormal behavior of the individuals. During this period nurses were given the responsibility of observing and reporting of patient's behavior and even to become co-therapist in these modes of behavioral modification.

Social science formulated that society is all cause of behavioral deviation in the individuals and society to be guided to help the individuals to correct the behavior. In this period nurses were asked to take up the responsibility of involving family members and society in treating and preventing the behavioral problems.

Psychiatrists started physical therapy in the treatment of their clients. Two main physical therapies were insulin coma therapy and the modified electroconvulsive therapy. After the insulin administration the patient slips into deep coma where the nurses were assigned to observe the vital signs and report if necessary. It happened while the patient is treated with unmodified electroconvulsive therapy also.

In 1950's, the psychotropic drugs entered in the psychiatic practices and nurses' role also changed accordingly. Here the nurse is supposed to know the chemical combination of the drug, routes of administration, dosage, indications, contraindications, side effects and nurses responsibilities when these drugs are administered.

The increasing number of individuals with behavioral problems in the world is great and alarming. The non-availability of enough hospital beds is a considerable problem of many countries. The policy makers in different countries shifted the focus of treating of these individuals from inpatient setup to out patient or to the community. National Mental Health Program (NMHP) was formulated and the community approach of psychiatry patients in practice. Accordingly, nurses' role also changed shifting from in patient setup to community. Therefore, she is involved at three levels of prevention, i.e. primary prevention, secondary prevention and tertiary prevention. In this context, Clifford Beers to be remembered. Having spent several years in mental hospital he wrote a book called "A Mind that Found Itself" in 1907. He emphasized on prevention and early recognition of behavioral changes.

Maxwell Jones demonstrated the practice of Milieu therapy and therapeutic community. Psychiatric nurses act as a team member in the procedure of Milieu therapy and therapeutic community.

There is one commendable development in psychiatric nursing itself without related to changes in psychiatric practice that is nothing but nursing process. The nursing process is an interactive problem solving process, a systematic and individualized way to fulfill the goal of nursing care. The nursing process acknowledges the autonomy of the individual and his freedom to make decisions and be involved in his own care. It is done in different interrelated phases.

Phases of Nursing process are:

1. Data collection.
2. Formulation of nursing diagnosis.
3. Planning the nursing care.
4. Implementation of nursing interventions.
5. Evaluation.

Practicing the nursing process is a definite forward step in nursing which make the nurse independent in her professional career.

To conclude the nursing started as a need based art. But developed tremendously with the help of the contributions from nursing leaders, enormous changes happened in medical practice, economy of different countries, policies of governmental and non governmental organizations and even the changes in bio and information technologies. It is not a simple art now. One should have required general education and prescribed professional education before she becomes a qualified nurse. To become psychiatric nurse she has to undergo a special training program by which she is able to perform the prescribed functions to look after the individuals in behavioral problems.

There are special courses conducted in different parts of the world to train the persons to become psychiatric nurse.

In India we have diploma courses conducted in:

1. NIMHANS Bangalore.
2. Raveli Ranchi.
3. Assam.

Postgraduate programs are available in:

1. NIMHANS Bangalore.
2. Chandigarh.

Around 1000 nurses have undergone DPN in NIMHANS and 30 nurses had postgraduation courses in NIMHANS (MSc).

TRENDS IN INDIA

In India, individuals with behavioral problems were admitted in the hospitals to avoid homicide in community. These indoors had only healthy, hefty male individuals to control their manic behavior.

Asylums were built here and there in India where nurses were given the responsibility of giving minimum physical care when they are alive and last rites after death.

In 1950s, trends in psychiatric care changed due to the drugs available in the practice of psychiatry and also other physical therapies made the nursing leaders to include some chapters in psychiatric nursing in nursing curriculum. The curriculum developed in 1986 by INC included a good amount of theory classes with practicals in nursing to care the individuals with behavioral problems. But in 1960, Normayil in Lucknow started the nursing training. Around this time, a training in psychiatric nursing started for 10 weeks, Later it is increased to 6 months.

In 1956, NIMHANS also started a program namely Diploma in Psychiatric Nursing (DPN) with maximum of 15 seats. It was discontinued for few years. But restarted in 1975 as a program for 11 months. Now it continues as a course for full academic years.

In 1975, RAK College of Nursing Delhi started postgraduation in psychiatric nursing. Later other colleges in the country like PGI Chandigarh, SNDT Bombay, CMC Vellore and NIMHANS also started Postgraduation in Psychiatric nursing.

At present 15 colleges give postgraduation in psychiatric nursing maximum of 60 seats.

DPN is offered in 3 institution with a maximum of 50 candidates.

Current Trends

Now, any medical or Paramedical course curriculum includes minimum exposure to psychiatry. Any branch of medicine and nursing concentrate on holistic approach. So, there is no question that psychiatric nursing is a speciality within nursing. All modern nursing theorems address the holistic nature of people and emphasize the need to care for a person's body and mind together. Now, the psychiatric nurse should keep her identity doing a better role. She can work at two levels. One, the nurse works with individual's families, communities and groups to promote health including mental health, assess dysfunction, assist clients to regain coping and prevent further disability. In the second level, the nurse can focus on full range of activities from mental health promotion to illness care, with additional skills in the diagnosis and treatment of mental disorders.

In addition to these levels of practice there are also clear subspecialities available by virtues of education or long-term experience. A few available subspecialities are child psychiatry, adolescent psychiatry, adult psychiatry, geriatric psychiatry, psychiatry for deaddiction and for depression and for chronically mentally ill. These categories are not virtually exclusive but they provide a means of identifying the nurses' specialization.

Future Directions

Psychiatric branch of medicine is moving towards biological, genetic and pharmacological era. These advances hold great promise for treatment. They have also raised concerns that advancing medical treatment could minimize the recognition of the continued need for psychotherapeutic interventions. So there is an urgent need for nurses with psychiatric nursing skills to provide service to individuals with acute and chronic illness terminal diagnosis, problem associated with ageing, grief, AIDS and other serious illness or stressful events.

Many believe that the major challenge for psychiatric nursing in the 21st century is keeping the nursing in par with the changes happening due to the new discoveries of science, genetics and technology. Psychiatric nursing must include neuroscience as well as behavioral sciences. The future provides challenging work for those interested in combining knowledge of neuroscience with an understanding of human behavior and their relationship to social and environmental conditions, affecting people.

Today many persons may be underdiagnosed and untreated. Those who are severely ill may be hospitalized for a limited period and get discharged with medication. So, there is an increased need for psychiatric specialists in home care. At the same time the motion of prevention is not being fully realized and practiced in most aspects of health. Mental health is not an exception to it.

So, it is important to have program to promote healthy parenting, stress reduction, avoidance of addictive substances in many communities, at large in all over the world. Contemporary issues such as domestic violence, addiction, homelessness, poverty where psychiatric care cannot remedy individual's problems, without solving or preventing larger social issue.

As the majority of nursing care moves from hospital to community there will be an increasing need for psychiatric nurses to use all of their creativities and skills to provide needed services in most effective way possible in community.

Closing down the hospitals, the government is looking for more and more homes for psychiatric patients. Nurses have many responsibilities in homes for these patients along with the home care responsibilities. Psychiatric nurses have to be closely vigilant to the changes happening around and prepare herself to meet the newer roles time to time.

CHAPTER 2

Mental Health and Mental Illness

INTRODUCTION

Health is defined as "A state of complete, physical, mental and social well-being not merely the absence of disease or infirmity—WHO.

This definition of health emphasizes the positive state of well-being rather than focusing on the lack of disease. People in their state of well-being or mental health, function comfortably within society and are satisfied with their achievements.

Mental health consists of multiple, various components, many of which are immeasurable by scientific standards. Further reason a concise, encompassing definition of mental health doesn't currently exists, although several definitions appear in the literature (Katherine and Patricia 2000).

Although there are several definitions they share a common core of meaning of mental health. Some emphasize on "Adjustment of individuals and some high light on 'effectiveness', 'satisfaction', subjective well-being, happiness, cheerfulness, etc.

Menninger defined mental health as, "the adjustment of human beings to each other and the world around them with a maximum of effectiveness and happiness."

Maslow studied a sample of real people whom he judged to be self-actualizing individuals (People moving in the direction of achieving their highest potentials) and considered them as mentally health individuals.

According to Maslow the self-actualized individual possess the following characteristics:

1. An appropriate perception of reality.
2. The ability to accept one's self, others and human nature.
3. The ability to manifest spontaneity.
4. The capacity to concentrate on problem solving.
5. A need for detachment and desire for privacy.
6. Independence, autonomy and resistance to enculturation.
7. An intensity of emotional reaction.
8. A frequency of 'Peak' experiences that validate the worthwhileness, richness and beauty of life.
9. An identification with human kind.
10. The ability to achieve satisfactory interpersonal relationship.
11. A democratic character structure and strong sense of ethics.
12. Creativeness.
13. A degree of non-conformance.

Indications for Good Mental Health

Jahoda (1958) identified a list of *six indicators for good mental health.*

1. A positive attitude towards self:

Person should have good feeling towards self. Accepts the strengths and limitations of self has a strong sense of personal identity and security in the environment.

2.Growth development and the ability for self-actualization

The person successfully achieves the tasks associated in each level of development and tries to achieve the highest level of his potentials.

3.Integration

Maintain an equilibrium or balance among various life processes.

4.Autonomy and self-determination

They have the abilities to perform as an independent and self-directed manner.

5.Perception of reality

Accurately reality perception is a positive indicator of mental health.

6.Environmental mastery and social competence

Individual achieves satisfactory role in group, society or environment. He or she is able to love and accept the love of others. Make proper decisions, adjust and adapt to situations. Has satisfaction in life.

Robinson (1983) defined Mental Health as "A dynamic state in which thought, feeling and behavior that is age appropriate and congruent with the local and cultural norms are demonstrated".

How to Spot Mentally Healthy People?

From various studies people have identified a number of characteristics, which are found in, people who are well-adjusted and who therefore, have healthy personalities. Few of them are as follows:

1. People who feel comfortable with other people by being able to:
   - Love themselves
   - Give love to others
   - Have lasting personal relationships
   - Respect the differences in people
   - Feel part of the group.
2. People who are able to handle the demands of life by:
   - Setting realistic goals for themselves
   - Planning ahead and not fearing the future
   - Cherishing experiences and welcoming new ideas
   - Being able to make their own decisions.
3. People who feel fulfilled in their lives by being able to:
   - Deal with most difficult situations
   - Accept their short-coming
   - Have self-respect
   - Take pleasure in simple everyday happenings.

Characteristics of a Mentally Healthy Individual

A mentally healthy individual:
1. Has ability to make adjustments.
2. Can remain unhampered by emotional conflict.
3. Has a philosophy of living and can confirm to and follow that philosophy.
4. Does not demonstrate any pathological symptomalotogy.
5. Finds satisfaction and fulfillment in exercising and expanding his potentials.
6. Can establish and maintain a meaningful relationship with others.

Tips to have Good Mental Health

- *In Order to have Good Mental Health one should have Good Physical Health*

Healthy food habits, adequate sleep, suitable physical exercises, yoga/meditation, early treatment of illness. Immunities are necessary to have good physical health. Healthy lifestyle is very essential to maintain good health.

- *Self-understanding*

In the world many people are interested to know about others rather than knowing about themselves. Knowing about others may result in feeling of inadequacy, inferiority and jealousy.

In order to be good we have to understand ourselves, positive and negative qualities, strength and weakness. So that we can strengthen the positive qualities and strive to overcome the negative qualities as much as possible.

- *Maintain Good Interpersonal Relationship with Others*

Healthy relationship offers real strength to our happiness. Harmonious relationship increases our well being whereas disharmony in relationship decreases the feeling of satisfaction with life.

- *Have a Confidential Relationship with one Person— Selected Friend, Counselor or a Relative*

It is scientifically proved that one of the effective ways of coping day-to-day tension is to share the feelings with others. 'Ventilating feeling' or sharing of the problems with others whom we have confidence is a healthy way. But selecting the person with whom one shares his problems one should be very careful. It cannot be done with anybody or everybody. It could be a professionally trained, counselor or good friend or life partner or a well-wisher in whom one has confidence. And also that person should have a balanced personality and experience in life to handle your problem. Or at least should be able to guide to proper person in case of he/she cannot solve the problem.

- *Have an Optimistic Outlook*

Optimistic outlook is very helpful in overcoming several problems in life. If one has optimistic outlook he can identify problem, analysis and perceives the problem in a different way. His reaction will be different to a person with pessimistic approach. If one has a pessimistic approach he cannot be happy at all. Neither too much optimism not too much pessimism but realistic optimism is very essential.

- *Avoid Unrealistic and High Expectations*

Most of the failures are due to unrealistic and high expectations, which cannot be achieved. So our goals need to be planned or revised to suit our capacities.

- *A Balance Schedule of Both Work and Play Leads a Happy Life*

A proportional mixture of work and recreation leads to happy life. Neither be workaholics nor be idlers.

- *Planning for the Future is a Part of Progressive means of Opportunity*

Mental Illness

A universal concept of mental illness is difficult owing to the cultural factors involved in the definition.

Horwitz (1982) identifies two elements they are:
1. Incomprehensibility.
2. Cultural relativity.

Incomprehensibility means inability of the general population to understand the motivation behind the behavior. When observers unable to find the meaning of the behavior they label the behavior as mental illness.

Culture relativity considers the rules, conventions and understanding of the behavior are cultural based. Behavior that is considered normal and abnormal is defined by ones cultural or social norms. Behavior viewed as normal may be considered abnormal in another culture.

Mental illness is characterized as "Maladaptive response to strenuous from the internal or external environment, evidenced by thoughts, feelings and behavior that are incongruent with the local and cultural norms, and interferes with the individual social, occupational or physical functioning".

The American Psychiatric Association (APA, 1994) defines mental disorder as "Clinically significant behavior or psychological syndrome or pattern that occurs in an individual and is associated with present distress (e.g., A painful symptom) or disability (i.e., impairment in one or more important areas of functioning) or with significantly increased risk of suffering death, pain disability or an important loss of freedom.

Mental health and mental illness are in a continuum. At a certain point in life any individual has the potential to move towards either side of the beam causing imbalance. Mental illness or normality is defined only in terms of the social norms.

Mental health———— Boderline Behavior ————→Mental illness

A person today may have good mental health. But due to various reasons, he comes to a point where he looses many characteristics of mental health when he is not able to balance with these stresses he slips into the state of mental illness.

As Joward emphasized "It is possible to be a normal personality and be absolutely miserable".

The person is considered normal by members of the social group if he plays his social role according to social expectation, but unless he deceives personal satisfaction from his role, he will likely in time develop a 'sick' personality. A person may look to be healthy when in reality he is sick. For example, when a person has headache but he camouflage his condition and behaves as a efficient alert and pleasant. The same is true of personality sickness. If a person is anxious, to be favorably judged by others can camouflage his feelings of inadequacy of martyrdom or of inferiority and behaves in such a manner as to create an impression that he is normal, well-adjusted person, understress. However, the camouflage often fails and the person reveals his real self. For example, selfish opportunists.

Thus, in every human being we find a combination of positive aspects and negative traits. The proportion may vary from person to person depending on the situation and life experiences one may be nearer to mental health or nearer to mental illness in the continuum.

CHAPTER 3

Principles of
Psychiatric Nursing

INTRODUCTION

Any professional organization or institution will have certain principles to be followed by its members. Nursing is not an exemptional to that. Any nurse has to have some basic principles and qualities while working with patient but a psychiatric nurse should have specific principles while practising her profession. The reason is many conditions in this branch has the symptoms of lacking insight of one self. Lack of insight is the main difference between these individuals and in general health and in these problems. Here the nurse is given special principles in psychiatry and in psychiatric nursing to deal with the situations in mental health hospitals community, etc. In the following pages of this chapter the special principles of psychiatric nursing are discussed.

Such principles are mentioned and discussed by Ruth Matheny and Mary Topalis in the year 1965. Other authors also discussed about the psychiatric nursing principles in their respective textbooks.

1. Accept the Patient Exactly as he is

Any unacceptable expressions of emotions like anger, violence, withdrawal, running away, abusing are only the symptoms of patient illness. These behaviors may be due to the change in his thought, feeling or actions.

So, nurse has to accept this behavior and convey the feeling that he is being loved, cared inspite of his behavior and try to establish rapport with the patient. Acceptance is also a part of providing a therapeutic environment which is emotionally neutral. This acceptance can be conveyed by the following:

a. *Being non-judgmental and non-punitive*: Any behavior of a psychiatric patient cannot be judged whether it is good or bad, right or wrong because he does it because of part of illness. You cannot tell it is right because it is not right. You cannot tell it wrong because it will hurt the feelings of the individual and it hinders, the establishment of rapport with the patient. It can be tactfully managed asking the individual to bring out other alternative way of doing the particular act.

   For example, patient A beats 'B' and claims that 'A' has done something great. The nurse does not tell it is right or wrong but ask the questions what do you think about it? Whether you have right to punish the individual 'B'? or report to the ward staff about 'B's? behavior • Individual. 'A' may comes out with the suggestions he could have reported 'B's behavior to ward staff. This type of discussions may give the insight to the individual 'A' or at least his attention can be diverted from the destructive behavior.

   Another way of handling this situation is the nurse working can say that "If I were in that situation I would have done this way". This also can give the individual 'A' a different thought and may modify the behavior in future.

As the nurse has no right to judge she has no right to punish as it is done for a normal individual. In psychiatric setup the punishment can be given by putting him in a single room (time out) ignoring his presence, withdrawing some facilities and cutting some incentives. These punishments are done as part of behavior modification. It will be effective when it is done along with the drug therapy.

b. *Show interest in patients as a person*: showing interest in patients is very important step in the development and maintenance of trusting relationship. This can be:
   - Shown by greeting them appropriately.
   - Asking the welfare, trying to fulfill his basic needs like personal hygiene, clothing, etc.
   - Trying to find out his likes and dislikes
   - Providing necessary items if possible
   - Explaining him when his demands are not meet in accepted manner.
   - Avoiding subjects which he does like.

c. Recognizing and reflecting feelings like anger, happiness and sadness and guilt, of patients to be recognized reflected back them. The feelings can be either by words or gestures the nurse should have the skill of identifying the feelings and reflect by asking questions accordingly.

For example, you seem to be sad today? What is worrying you?

You seem to be angry? What made you angry? Any event or any person?

When you reflect on their feelings it shows that you are genuinely interested in him.
   - You are giving him a chance to ventilate his feelings.

- The ventilation itself provides therapeutic effectiveness.

d. *Talk with a purpose*: Aimless conversation should be avoided while taking care of individual with behavior problems.

   Nurse should be aware of four stages of inter-personnel relationships which overlapse definitely. So, while talking with patient the nurse should be aware that in which stage of IPR she is. She should aim to achieve the objectives of that stage of IPR. But the same time she has to consider all psychiatric nursing principles.

   By this purposeful conversation patients day to day problems can be managed and also the nurse can achieve her goal of IPR.

e. *Listening:* Is an art needed for every walk of life as father, as a mother, as a teacher, as an administrator, as a nurse you should be a good listener. It is an essential quality required for psychiatric nurse also. Listening helps the person to ventilate the feelings which has a therapeutic effect. When patient starts communicating she should be a silent listener with non-directive and brief comment showing interest in what patient is saying.

f. *Permit patient to ventilate strongly held feelings:* Unexpressed strong emotions are always dangerous. So psychiatric nurse should permit to express the strongly held feelings without dis-approval or punishment. Patient can be permitted to express his feelings not only in words but action also, without distinctly the men or material.

   For example, Pillow or boxing board can be given where the patient can hit or beat to express his angry feelings.

The relief of strongly held expressions can lesson the tension and anxiety which makes the patients relax.

2. Self-understanding is a Therapeutic Tool.

Self-understanding is a necessary quality for a psychiatric nurse. Any behavior by a nurse has a positive or negative effect on the patient will have hindrance in achieving goal.

So person uses different ways to deal with it. According to Colman different mental mechanisms are used by individual to achieve their goal. Other psychologists tell people behave differently when there are hindrances to achieve the goal. One group put more effort others use different means. Yet other will change the goal when they realize that it cannot be achieved. But there are groups to use extreme step to achieve the goal by distinctioning himself or others.

The nurse can introspect herself to which group she belongs. She also can modify her behavior which is acceptable in the community. When she does the introspection she can understand herself better. This self-understanding can be used while she take care of mentally ill-patients.

When she is dealing with psychiatric patients. When she confronts with patients problem, she introspects and use different ways to solve the problems. It can be putting more effort, or using different means or changing the goal. But make sure either herself or patients should not use any methods which may be harmful to them or others.

Nurses feeling, reactions or handling the problems should not have adverse effect on patients and patient problems.

This self-understanding can be nourished by:
- Exchanging personal experiences with other team members
- Participating in group conference, regarding patients care
- Evaluating her own behavior with the peer group
- Introspecting everyday her actions in the working area by asking questions why did I feel and act the way I did today?

3. Be Consistent While Working with Patients with Behavior Problem

Consistency means same action to be followed. Consistency should be in the individual nurse itself, among the nurses of different shifts among the nurses of different cadre and among the other team members.

The consistency also should be in the ward routine, attitudes towards patients, limitations put in the patient, concessions and facilities given, visiting time, persons and Do's and Don'ts, etc.

This is achieved by giving proper orientation at the time of admission, giving the activity schedule of the ward, giving the instructions any other rules and regulations while the patient is in the ward. Introduction to nurses and other team members also necessary. This will reduce the patient's anxiety and will know when to do and what to do while patient is in the ward.

Consistency can be achieved only when every individual of the treating team work together in the all above said areas. Then only patients emotional security can be achieved at maximum level.

4. Reassurance to be given in an Acceptable and Realistic Manner

Reassurance is giving support and building the confidence in the patient. It should be in a realistic manner without giving the false assurances.

Avoid statements like:

- You will get well
- Your fears are groundless
- You take up a better job
- You will pass with good marks.

Reassurance can be given by:

- Being near to the patient seen if the patient is not talking
- Listening to patient without showing surprise or disapproval
- Not arguing or not contradicting
- Accepting his feelings as it is
- Doing things to him without expecting any returns
- Be truly interested in patient problems.

5. Patients Behavior can be Changed Through Emotional Experience not by Rational Interpretation

Many individuals with behavioral problem do not have the reasoning ability. They go with their feelings. So, to correct their behavior reasoning may not be helpful. They have to be corrected only by providing the needed experience of feelings, role play, sociodrama, transactional analysis are few methods of creating emotional experience in such patients.

6. Avoid Unnecessary Increase in Patients Anxiety

Anxiety is a feeling of fear of unknown object or event. It is a feeling of apprehension.

Anxiety is the basic problem in causation of behavioral problems. So, already mentally ill people will have some amount of anxiety.

This anxiety is not only due to disease process but also due to separation from the family, new atmosphere, stigma attached to the diseases, poor prognosis, etc. So, nurse should be very careful not to increase the anxiety level of the patient but try to decrease the anxiety.

- Not projecting her own anxiety and apprehension on patients
- Giving orientation to the physical structure of the ward co-patients team members rules and regulations, policies activity and schedules, etc.
- Not contradicting patients psychiatric ideas
- Not using professional terms while talking to patients
- Avoiding careless conversations within patients hearing about his personal life
- Being sincere to the patient
- Not demanding to me complete the task, which cannot be met by me
- Not showing indifference and negligence.

7. Observe Objectively to Understand and Interpret the Patients Behavior

Continuous close observation is the most important function of the psychiatric nurse. This must be objective observation. This helps to interpret the behavior and avoid untoward incidences. They help to record patients' behavior which helps to communicate patients' behaviors to other disciplinary team members.

This objective observation can be interpreted well by the previous experience of the nurse and patients' history and other records and reports of the patient. The skill also can be developed daily by observing and putting the question "why" this behavior from "this patients"? This helps to know the specific reasons for the behavioral problems in the particular patient.

If your interpretation is wrong ask the question "Why" and also take help from others to understand.

Objective observations can be affected adversely by:
- Judging the patients behavior right or wrong
- Having pre-conceived ideas about the patient
- Justifying or defending nurse herself
- Pre-occupation of nurses own problem.

8. Maintain Realistic Nurse-Patients Relationship

The relationship between the nurse and patient should be only professional, not personal one. This relationship to be oriented to patients' needs but not the nurses needs. Nurse should analyze periodically the interaction between herself and the patient and able to differentiate between patients demand and actual needs. She also should be aware of different stages of IPR and plan for the limitation phase. Once the working phase is finishing she should be able to prepare the patient for discharge and to lead a independent life without her assistance. To keep a healthy professional realistic relationship nurse may have to avoid:
- Meeting the patients out of duty hours
- Taking the patients for restaurant
- Giving and taking gifts
- Giving special considerations.

9. Verbal and Physical Force must be Avoided if Possible

As accepted the patients as it is the main principle of psychiatric nursing, the nurse cannot use any punishments whether is verbal or physical. Any forceful verbal directions, or abusive and bad language will not be helpful to the patient to change his behavior unless he comes in touch with reality. So, it should be avoided.

Physical force also should be prevented unless it is very necessary such as homicidal, suicidal, assaultive behavior. If at all physical force is used it should be done quickly firmly and in well-planned manner.

For example, If the patients is violent, not able to be controlled. Patient can be carried to a place by adequate staff members and given parental medication in shortest time. No verbal comments during this time or anger of any kind to the patients is shown. Patient should not be reminder of this incident as kind of punishments.

In occasions when the patient are unmanageable they can be isolated in single room. This isolation can help them to relax and come out of their dangerous behavior and even modify their behavior later. The patient should be informed about this when he can understand this made of treatment.

10. Nursing Care Centered on Patient as a Person, not on Control of Symptoms

Now, it is the era of holistic approach as is happening in any branch of medicine it is applicable in psychiatric nursing also. Treatment or the management should not be symptom centered. The nurse should be able to identify different causes for this particular symptom in the particular patient whether its is due to physical psychological, financial, social occupational or any other. So, the management also should be directed towards the causes after getting enough evidence for the cause.

For example, In a child psychiatry center there may be three children having hysterical convulsion. Each may have different causes for their convulsion. One may be reacting to a strict parenting, who expect the child to get first rank always, one may be reacting to abusive and assaultive teacher in the school yet other may be reacting to parent who is more attached to other sibling in the family. The nurse should be able to identify the cause and able to rectify the cause with the help of parents and other concerned people.

11. Routines and Procedures Explained at Patients Level of Understanding

Things are changing very fast in all dimensions. People are aware of their rights and privileges. The psychiatric nurses should be careful as they can be sued for any least negligence from their side. They may overlook patients ability to understand the routine and procedures done on them. But it is not so. Though they are mentally ill they should be considered as any other sick person. So, it is essential that nurse has to explain the procedures and the ward routine to the patients according to the level of understanding. It is one of the rights of the mental-ill individual.

This explanation can reduce patients' anxiety and helps developing therapeutic interpersonal relationship.

12. Positive Reinforcement to be used wherever is Possible.

Self-esteem is an important drive for a healthy living. Many of the patients who come to psychiatric setup will have reduced self-esteem at various degrees. Improving esteem is one of the essential component of psychiatric nursing.

During her daily activities the nurse has to recognize and reflect the positive things in patients' life and reinforce the same. It is a reward for his positive act, with this he may make it as a habit which will indirectly increase his self-esteem:

For example:

- *When a depressed patient starts working in the ward the nurse says "I am happy to see your working or its good to find a change in you".*
- *When a withdrawn child comes for the play voluntarily the nurse says "I am happy to see you in the playground it is good". I hope you will continue. So, child will feel happy and will be active in the group later when she is accepted in the group naturally the self-esteem of the child will be increased.*
- *Any other activities like, bathing, brushing, combing hair, coming to activity or therapy group can be recognized and reinforced.*

Reinforcements are of various types like: Psychological, physical and financial, etc.

The common reinforcement used are:

- Words of appreciation
- Words of acceptance
- Patting
- Giving eatables or cash
- Providing some privileges like seeing TV, talking for outing, etc.

Nurses are the first persons who observe the positive action in the patient behavior so she should act immediately without delay in giving reinforcements to have maximum effect.

13. Structured Activity Schedule as a part of Psychiatric Nursing

Each area of psychiatric ward should have a activity schedule from morning to night. It can be like personal hygiene, prayer, exercises, group work, interactivity, recreation, social therapy, work therapy, religious activities, etc.

The advantages of schedule activities are:
- It reduces patients' anxiety as he knows what is to be done next?
- It reduces the hallucination and delusions
- Keep the patient awake and active in the day which helps in good night sleeps
- It helps in preventing self-injury and hazardous behaviors
- It helps in observing the patients', his interest and disinterest in activities
- It helps occupational therapist to find a placement for the patients
- It helps to have increased self-esteem
- Reduces obsessions and compulsions.

14. Many Procedures are Modified but Basic Principles Remain Unaltered.

All the nursing procedure like parental injections dressing enemas, rhyles tube feedings are same as for other physically ill-patients. But it will be modified according to the situation without changing the basic principles of the procedure.

1. *For example, To the excited patients the injection is given in a place where the patient is.*
2. First few days of admission even interview can be done wherever her patient is 15. Rehabilitation should be planned from the 1st day itself. It can be in the form of occupational placement, residential placement, half way hornes, sheltered workshop, etc.

BIBLIOGRAPHY

1. Mary Varghese issue Essentials of Psychiatric and Mental Health Nursing BI Churchill Living stone New Delhi 1994.
2. Matheney and Topalies 1956.
3. Ms. K. Lalitha—'Mental health and psychiatric Nursing' Gajanana book publishers 1995.
4. Stuart W. Gail (1998) Pocket guide series—Psychiatric nursing V edition Mosby Co.

CHAPTER 4

History Taking and Mental Status Examination in Psychiatric Nursing

INTRODUCTION

The correct diagnosis in general medicine depends upon the careful history taking and clinical examination. The history taking in psychiatry and psychiatric nursing differs from the rest of the branches of medicines and surgery. Here the history taking is not only to obtain the history but also to elicit the clinical signs. For that reason one should remember that the interviewing of an individual with behavioral problems is a practical skill which can be achieved only through carrying out interviews under the supervision or watching experienced interviewers at work.

Why history taking in psychiatry and psychiatric nursing is different?

It is because of few reasons:

First of all the patient may not have the insight to express the problems. If a person experiences fever or pain anywhere in the body he reports it. But a psychiatric patient especially with psychotic conditions never considers that he has some problem. So, the history in detail only will help a clinician to elicit the signs and make the diagnosis.

Next problem in this field is the stigma attached to behavioral problems. There are chances that either the patient or the relatives try to hide the signs and their duration. The gradual onset of certain conditions also makes the individual and relatives to overlook the symptoms.

Another important point to remember in this area is that no absolute measurement tool is available in this field. Therapist or interviewer makes the diagnosis subjectively than objectively. In general, medicine thermometer is there to measure temperature, sphygmomanometer is there to record the blood pressure, different scanning machines are available to visualize the internal organs accurately. But in psychiatric nursing the detail history taking and continuous close observations on the behavior only can make good diagnosis.

Whenever possible the history should be from the patient. The information should be supplemented or confirmed by a close relative or friend who stays with the patient for a considerable duration.

History should be taken systematically and in the same order to ensure that important aspects are not forgotten and also to make easy for other team members to refer the notes. We know the importance of history taking and also the need for a scheme for the same.

A Scheme for History Taking

1. Identification of patient: Identification of the patient name, age, sex educational status, marital status, occupation, state of origin, mother tongue, nationality, etc.
2. *Informant* Name, relationship to the patient, length of acquaintance. Interviewers view about the reliability of the information.

3. *Source of referral if any*
4. *History of present complaints*
   - Complaints are listed in chronological order with duration
   - Complaints are described in sentences as they occurred in details
   - Any treatment given, its details and effect
   - Any other physical complaints at present or in the past. If so treatment taken
   - Negative history
5. *Family history:* Genogram is drawn minimum for 2 generations.

   - Male is denoted as
   - Female
   - Death   X
   - Disease   ///

Consanguineous marriage is denoted with double line.

Abortion or stillbirth is denoted with short lines and small figures.

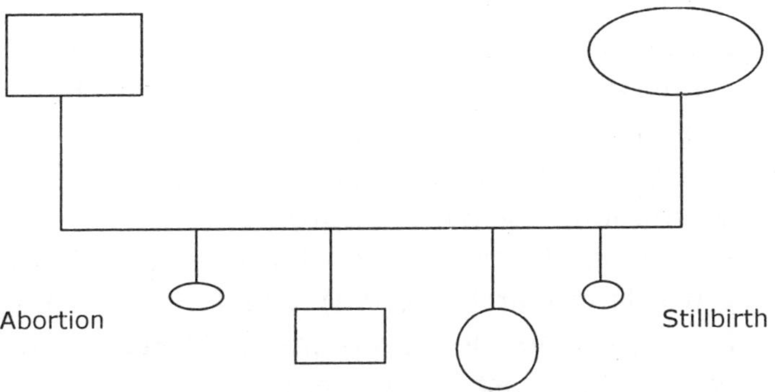

Remarriage is denoted on either side with a different line.

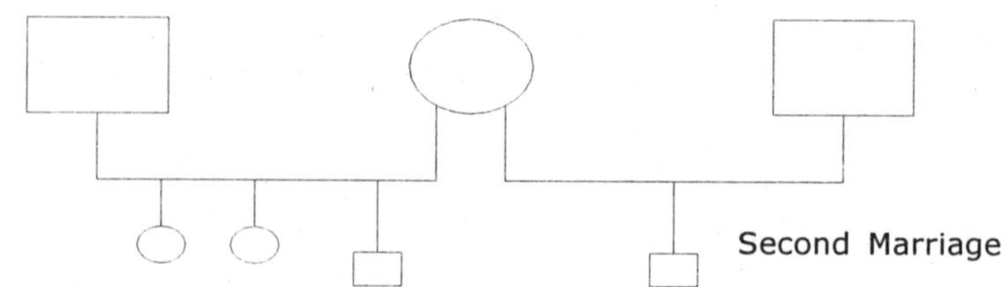

After Genogram

Mother-age educational status, occupation, relationship with patient.
Father-age, educational status, occupation, relationship with family members especially with patient.
Siblings 1.
      2.
      3.

6. *Personal history*
   a. Problems during antenatal period natal and immediate postnatal period.
   b. Milestones-if abnormal details.
   c. *Preschooling*: Behavior any special health problems.
   d. *Schooling:* Age of starting of schooling, behavior; scholastic performance completion of schooling, Higher education details.
   e. *Occupation:* Chronology, performance, salary, promotion, discipline, awards.
   f. *Menstrual history:* Age of menarche, attitude towards monarch (period), regularity, amount of flow dysmenorrhea, premenstrual tension, age of menopause, last menstural period.
   g. *Marital history:* Age of marriage, mode of marriage, relationship with spouse.

h. *Sexual history:* Attitude, homosexual, hetero sexual, multiple partners.
i. *Children:* Normal, age, abortions, stillbirth, temperament, emotional stability, physical and mental development.
j. *Personality:*
   - Premorbid personality, with family members, friends, colleagues.
   - How spends the leisure time
   - Mood
   - Habits.

7. *Mental status examination:*
   a. General
   b. Non-cooperative patient
   c. Unconscious patient.

Mental status examination is an important component of history taking. It should be done systematically. During this process and positive finding are observed, it should be written in detail. MSE is to be repeated several times during the course of illness. It will help to know changes in the symptoms, to know the effectiveness of treatment symptoms. Mental status examinations for a conscious, patient is done under the following heading:

i. *General appearance.* This included the whether the patient,
   - Ill or well,
   - Clean or unclean
   - Tense or relaxed
   - Cooperative/uncooperative
   - Eye contact is adequate or not.
   - Hesitate to come inside the interview room or voluntarly coming inside
   - Any ties or mannerism present
   - Any catatonia phenomenas or not, look anxious or not.

ii. *Psychomotor activity*
   Whether the psychomotor activities increased, decreased or normal whether the walk is slow or fast or any other abnormal activity like jumping, running, talking continuously wishing repeatedly or any other unusual activity.

iii. *Speech*
   - Is the speech poor or excessive
   - Is the speech continuous or only answers to the questions
   - Whether the tone is low or high
   - Is the tempo fast or slow (Tempo is the speed)
   - Is the reaction time normal or delayed
   - Is it relevant to the questions, time and situation
   - Description of speech can be under the heading of:
     - Relevance, coherence, volume, tone, tempo, reaction time, etc.

iv. *Thought*
   Thought is examined under the headings of:
   Form and stream
   - Is there any flight of ideas?
   - Is there any retardation of thinking?
   - Is there circumstantiality?
   - Is there preservation?
   - Is there any thought block?

   Possession
   - Is there obsession?
   - Is there compulsion?
   - Is there any thought alteration?
   - If there is obsession further details should be collected like, nature, ideas, doubts, imaginary, impulses and phobias.

- If there is compulsions record the action of compulsions and also whether a under control or yielding to compulsion.

Content

- Is there any delusions?
- If there is, it is single or multiple?
- Is it grandiose, persecutory, nihilistic?
- Is the delusion well systematized?
- Is the delusion poorly systematized?
- Are there any worries, preoccupation, hypo-chondriacally?
- Is there any ideas of worthlessness, guilt, hopelessness, suicidal ideas?

v. *Mood*

- Mood is assessed by looks subjective and objective
- Is it longitudinal (mood) or cross-sectional (affect)?
- It also assessed under the heading of quality of emotion (happiness, anxiety).
  - Depth of emotion, Ranges of affective response, diurnal variation of liability—(rapid change of mood).
- Question can be:
  - What is your mood like?
  - How are you in your spirit?
  - How you thought that life is not worth living?
  - Have you ever thought of ending your life?
  - Have you attempted to end your life?
  - Are you experiencing any palpitation, dry mouth, sweating, trembling?
  - Is he looking blunt, cheerful?

vi. *Perception*

- Is there illusions or hallucination?
- If it is, record the modalities, visual, auditory, smell, touch, taste, pain, deep sensation.

- Are they verbal, non-verbal, continuous or intermittent, whether it is 1st persons, 2nd person or 3rd person, whether it commanding, pleasant, unpleasant imaging or pseudo?

vii. *Cognitive functioning*

- This includes several factors. They are:
  a. Orientation to person, place and time is assessed asking questions like the name of place where he is, time of the interview and person doing interview or person who accompanied.
  b. *Attention and concentration*
     This test includes:
     The digital span test: Patient is given the following instruction:
     I will be saying, some digits, listen carefully, when I finish you have to repeat them in the same order.
     For example,   5-3,7
     1-5,8,7
     1,6,4,95

It may be up to 8 digit. So it can be recorded that the patient could tell how many digits?

Backward digital span can be used where the patient is asked to tell the serial backward, i.e. if the interview tells 7,6 the patient has to tell 6,7.

Serial Substraction

- The patient is to tell the number in reversed order *For example, (1) 20 to 0*
- In reversed order in 15 seconds, *for example, (2) 40-37 series 10 seconds.*
- 100-y 10, 93, 86. In 120 seconds

The series of 7 from 100 can be asked that 100, 93, 86 so on. The time given for this is 120 seconds.

Memory

This includes immediate, recent and remote memory.

Immediate It can be tested by digital span.

Recent Tested by address test.

Any new address is said and talk to the patient any other matter. After 3 to 5 minutes ask the patient to repeat the address. Write exactly what the patient could tell.

Remote Memory

Date of birth, number of children, family members and any other relevant incidences in life.

Intelligence

- For literate individuals
  - Name of Prime Minister
  - Capital of the countries

For illiterates

- Seasons
- Crops and fruit
- Prices of grain
- Prices of lands

Comprehension

The ability to understand the questions asked during interview.
Few examples are:
- What you will do when you miss a train while you are on a journey?
- What you will do when you feel cold?

Arithmetic

Simple adding, subtracting can be asked. Even some division also can be asked.

Abstraction

Abstraction is tested by asking the similarities and difference of articles, animals, etc.
Similarities between:
- Orange and banana
- Dog and lion
- Eye and ear
- North and west.

Differences can be asked, e.g.,
- Potato and stone
- Cinema and radio
- Fly and butterfly.

Proverbs and the meanings also been asked to assess the abstractions.
- A barking dog never bites
- Empty vessels make more noise.

Judgment
- Personal
- Social
- And test.

Social Judgment is assessed by the behavior in social situations.

Test judgment is usually asking the question.

1. If the home you are in catches fire what you will do?
2. If you find a stamped envelop sealed and addressed what you will do?

Mental status examination (MSE) can be repeated is a day if needed is acute stage of illness later it can be daily.

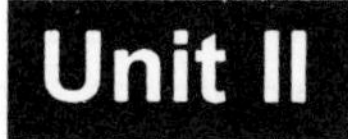

CHAPTER 5

Causes and Classification of Mental Illness

INTRODUCTION

The other word for psychiatric illness is abnormal behavior or deviated behavior.

What is deviated behavior? When person behaves in a way that he is not expected to behave in that manner in that particular situation, it is called deviated behavior or abnormal behavior, which is called as psychiatric illness. This explanation also is very vague and subjective. Because a particular behavior of an individual can be accepted by certain people in the community and others may not accept it. So, there are reports of abnormal behavior of individuals especially of great leaders in history like Nero Ceasar the emperor of Rome (who finally committed suicide), Hitlor of Germany, Tippu Sultan of Indian origin. But never anybody identified them as having behavioral problems or given any treatment. When you look at the early history of medicine the individuals behaved abnormally were driven out of the society because they believed it is caused by demon or evil sprits which will affects the other members of the family. Other reason was, they considered that these individuals will harm themselves and others. The influence of evil sprits in these individuals is only a superstition not a cause of mental illness. Later society noticed some changes in individual with behavioral problems according to the changes happened in the moon. That is the full moon day and a moonless day, there were absolute visible changes in the behavior of these individuals. This fact also is considered as superstition as there is no scientific evidence that moon has something to do with an individuals with behavioral problems.

It came a long way that Fraud the father of psychology contributed his views about the causes of behavioral problems. Fraud (1961) identified the human development by stages. He considered the first 5 years of child's life be the most important, as he believes that all individuals basic character had been formed by the age of five.

Sociologists refer that society influences the individuals behavior. But in the medical model the etiology of behavioral problems is enlightened as the imbalances of neurochemical substances which is otherwise called neurobiological model. This indirectly talking about the genetic possibility of behavioral problems. After the above said discussions the probable causes of behavior deviation can be as follows:

The present day it is believed that no organisms can cause mental illness but possible causes are:

1. Genetic theories.
2. Neurochemical theories.
3. Neuroendocrinal theories.
4. Psychosocial theories.
5. Personality theories—psychological theories.
6. Neuropathological theories.

Genetic Theories

Genetic can be proved by different studies like segregation studies (pedegree), family studies, twin studies and adoption.

Neurochemical Theories

Where the investigation are done to see the level of neurochemical substances in different conditions. The definite pattern is still under scrutiny. But it is definite that there is an imbalance of neurochemical substances in these individuals. Which are corrected with the drugs which contain these substances. Why these imbalances? Is it because of inherited properties of brain and because is it the influence of environment or is it because of the experience of the individual during his first 5 years of his life? All these questions are not answered authentically.

Neuroendocrinal Theories

As we know the genetic factors has a definite influence in the endrocrine system of the individual. The endocrinal system has a direct influence of the individual's behaviors. In other words' the endocrine balance and imbalances can cause behavioral balance and imbalance in an individual.

Psychosocial Theories

This is a combination of psychological and social theories. Here Fraud can be remembered who talks about the experience in childhood which may be the cause of abnormal behavior in later stage of life. He also talks about the learning theories, which can influence the behaviors of an individual. To say in simple words here the theory tells that any behavior which is rewarded in the early life will be continued in adolescent and adulthood—irrespective of the action is good or bad. On the other side, any action in the childhood which is not rewarded or punished will be discontinued in later stages of life. So, what is learnt as good or bad may continue in the adulthood which is called the learning theory of behavioral problem.

Personality Theories

Few studies tell that particular personalities are prone to get some particular behavior deviations. But one look at the behavioral problems, of individuals and their earlier personalities 'many times they do not correlate. Still few reports are quoted below.

Kraeplen (1921) suggested that people with cyclothemic personalities (that is those with repeated and sustained mood change) were more prone to develop manic-depressive disorder. Leonharsl et al (1962) reported the association to be stronger among patients with bipolar disorders than among those with unipolar disorders. But if the personality is assessed without knowing the illness, the bipolar patients were not found to have cyclothemic personality traits.

The individuals with an ankastic personality (Khan 1928) are liable to develop anxiety and depression disorders. Avoidence personality can lead to depressive behaviors. But how these individuals develop these personalities? The answer is it can be due to

Heriditory and genetic factors

Enviornmental factors

Family factors

Experiences in early childhood

So the personality theories cannot be counted as a separate place in the causes of mental disorders. But it is a factor, which contributes in the enhancement of behavioral problems.

Neuro-Pathological Theories

This theory talks about that any structural changes of the brain can cause behavioral changes. In some condition like schizophrenias and affective disorders do not show any structural changes in the brain according to the postmortem studies. But the postmortem studies suggest that the theories of the mamillary bodies in the brain are seen in the individuals who had amnesic syndrome or profound disorders of memory.

It is to be remembered that the behaviors of the children with microcephaly, macrocephaly or hydrocephalus is expected to be abnormal according to degree of the structural changes in the brain. So, is it not the structural change—a cause of behavioral deviation?

As it is discussed earlier the causes of abnormal behaviors are closely interlinked. A single psychiatric disorder may result from several causes. For that reason a different scheme of classification is required. An acceptable approach is to divide the causes chronologically into predisposing, precipitating and perpetuating.

PREDISPOSING FACTORS

These are the factors which include genetic, environment *in utero*. Physical, psychological and social factors in the infancy and childhood. Some writers talk about constitution which includes physical and psychological structure of the individual. It may be only restricted to childhood or may be of adolescent and early adulthood.

PRECIPITATORY FACTORS

These are some of the event which occur first before the occurrence of illness. It may be physical and social. *For example, cerebral tumor or drugs used for any other disease which can be considered as physical, Loss of job or sudden loss of loved ones. Financial loss can be considered as a social problem.* Sometimes both physical and social factors can trigger an abnormal behaviors.

For example, a head injury can cause physical abnormality (structural changes in the brain) and social problems of finance or disfigurement of body. So, any stressful event can be the preceding cause of abnormal behavior.

PERPETUATING FACTORS

Once the disorder occurs. There are some factors which can prolong the disorder or perpetuate it.

For example, once the illness occurs the individual may be terminated from the job or dishonored in the society which may act as a secondary cause of the illness. The individual also may show the symptoms of depression or withdrawal which can further activate the condition. When the treatment is planned it should be a holistic approach to prevent or treat the perpetuating factors.

No single theory is self-explanatory or can be accepted unopposed as it can be questioned by an experienced observer in the psychiatric field.

The recent term to express the etiology of psychiatric illness is biopsychophysiological theory. The process which produce consciousness rely on the complexities of brain anatomy and the principles of neurophysiology. Here comes the concept of neurons which receives the input from different part of body and the neurons ability to discharge the excretory or inhibitory stimuli which is released in the synaptic cleft, along with the neurotransmitters. So, genetic theory is more strong when we consider the theories of psychiatric illness. The coming days have to prove whether it is strong or strongest.

CLASSIFICATION

Classification systems provide language by which to define, describe, and record phenomena and allow health

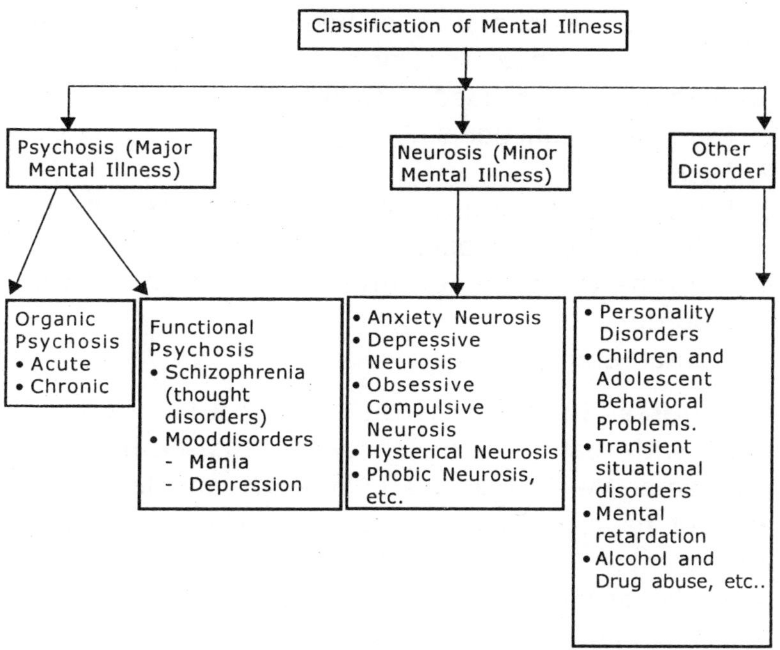

professionals to document the differences and similarities between condition. In general medicine, the classification is easy because usually the conditions are fairly straight forward. But in psychiatry very few disorders have an indisputable etiology but most can be classified only on symptoms. So, classification are needed in psychiatry in order that professionals can communicate easily about the nature of patient's problems and prognosis and treatment.

Around 3000 years ago Ayurvedic system of medicine classified mental illness as *vatonmada, kaphonmada, pitonmada*, etc. But Allopathic system tried to classify mental illness around 120 years ago. Some more and more professionals from different parts of the world participated in the whole process. The work has gone through several major drafts each prepared by national and international psychiatric faculties. In ICD 10 chapter Vth (F) givens the classification of psychiatric problem.

For the understanding of beginners, in profession or for a common man, the psychiatric illness or behavioral problems can be divided as follows:
1. Psychosis: Functional + organic.
2. Neurosis.
3. Behavioral problems in children and adolescent—it is still a matter of debate.
4. Personality disorder and transient situational disorders.
5. Mental retardation.

Psychosis In psychosis the individual is lacking the touch with reality. He never realizes that he has some problems. He creates his own world and lives in it, without having, realization about the normal existing environment. He gets stimuli according to his inner-self and believes they are real. He experiences hallucinations, delusions, illusion and act accordingly.

TYPES OF PSYCHOSIS

Functional Psychosis

It can be divided into affective psychosis—mania, depression (unipolar or bipolar).

Psychosis where thoughts are more prominent, e.g. schizophrenia.

Mania Depressive Disorder

One term expresses the swing of mood of the individual from one extreme to the other. But often it is seen that over the years of episodes of attack in individuals, one mood remains predominant during the illness. So, manic depressive illness may be further classified into mania type or depressive type + or it may be called bipolar affective disorder, when both mania and depression come at different time in life.

This is a figurative representation of manic type of psychosis.

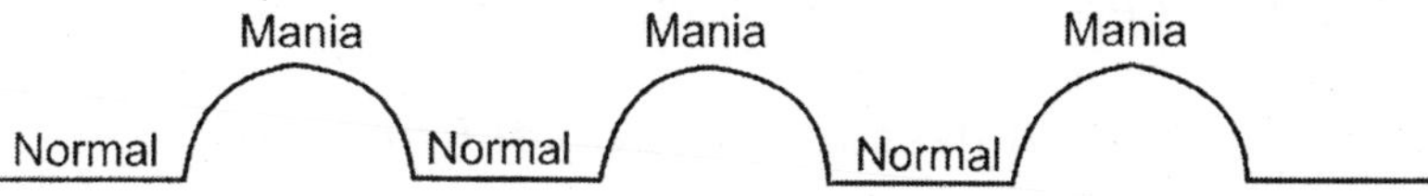

This is a figurative representation of depressive type of psychosis.

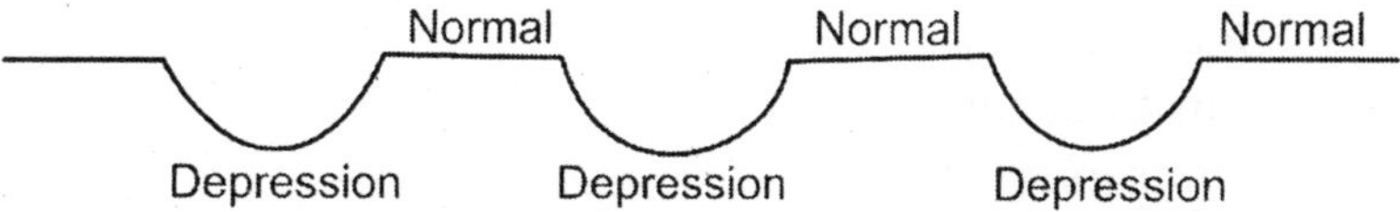

This is a figurative in presentation of BAPD (Bipolar affective psychotic disorder).

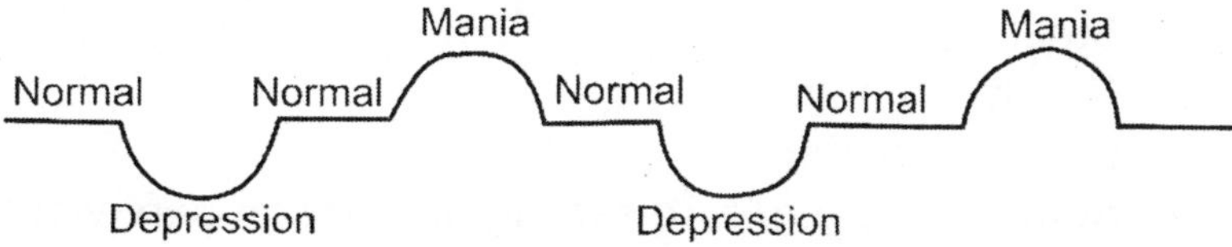

Psychosis other than affective disorders are called schizophrenia.

Schizophrenia is divided into the following:

- i.   Simple schizophrenia
- ii. Hebephronic schizophrenia
- iii. Catatonic schizophrenia
- iv. Paranoid schizophrenia

Neurosis

In neurosis there is gross disturbance in reality orientation. This disorder may be an outcome of either the individual's experience in infancy and early childhood or the stress for current environmental factors. They use defense mechanism to cope with the conflict and anxiety.

The disease conditions are anxiety neurosis conversion disorders, phobic disorders, obsessive, compulsive neurosis, depressive neurosis, etc.

Children and Adolescent Behavioral Problems

a. *Emotional disorders*
   - School refusal
   - Feeding problem
   - Bed wetting
   - Somatisation
b. *Conduct disorders*
   - Stubburness
   - Temper tantrums
   - Demanding
   - Stealing
   - Cruelty to animals
   - Drug adduction
   - Aggression, e.g. fore setting distruction behavior.
c. *Attention deficits and hyperacture behavior*
   - Impulsion....
   - Distractability
d. *Pervasive disorders*
   - Autism
   - Reciprocal social interaction
   - Repetative sterio type activities.

Personality Disorder, Transient Situational Disorders

a. *Impulsive*
   - Hetronic
   - Boarderline
   - Antiapatory.
b. *Anxions*
   - Avoidance
   - Dependant
   - Passive Aggressive.

c. *Peculiar*
- Odd and mixed and not been able to categorise.

Mental Retardation

- Mild
- Moderate
- Severe
- Proforced.

The existing two systems of classifications are: DSM (Diagnostic Statistical Manual) and ICD (International classification of diseases. DSM classified and modified it four times. The present one which is in use is DSM IV-R. The system of ICD did revision for several times and present systems is called ICD-10. Every revision was done according to the experience of professionals.

Classification according to ICD-10*

F00-F09:   *Organic, including symptomatic and mental disorders*
This group includes mental and behavioral disorders which have a demonstratable and independently diagnosable cerebral diseases. This disorder includes dementia of various kinds and delirium organic mental disorders.

F10-F19:   *Mental and behavioral disorders due to psychoactive substance use*
This group includes problems due to use of alcohol opiods cannabis, sedatives and other psychoactive substances. It also includes acute intoxication, harmful use, dependence syndrome, withdrawal state, etc.

F20-F29:   *Schizophrenia, schizotypal and delusional disorders*

*From-The ICD-10 classification of mental and behavioral disorders World Health Organisation, Geneva 1992

This group has the problems charachterized by disturbances of thought perception affect, etc. Disorders in this group are schizophrenia, schizotypal disorder, persistent delusional disorders, acute and transient psychotic disorders, induced delusional disorder, schizo affective disorders.

F30-F39: *Mood (affective) disorders*

This group includes mental and behavioral disorders characterized by disturbance of mood. The disorders included here are manic episode, bipolar affective disorder, depressive episode, recurrent depressive disorder, Persistent mood (affective) disorders, etc.

F40-F48: *Neurotic, stress-related and somatoform disorders.*

This group includes mental and behavioral disorders which are labeled as neurotic disorders with emphasis on psychological reasons. The disorders in this section includes: Phobic anxiety disorders, other anxiety disorders, obsessive/compulsive disorder, reaction to severe stress and adjustment disorders, dissociative (conversion) disorders, somatoform disorders, other neurotic disorder

F50-F59: *Behavioral syndromes associated with physiological disturbances and physical factors.*

This disorder in this section includes eating disorders, nonorganic sleep disorders, sexual dysfunction, not caused by organic disorder or disease, disorders associated with the puerperium, abused of non-dependence-producing substances.

F60-F69: *Disorders of adult personality and behavior*
The disorders in this section include, specific personality disorders, mixed and other personality disorders, enduring personality changes, not attributable to brain damage and disease, habit and impulse disorders, gender identity disorder, disorder of sexual preference, other disorders of personality.

F70-F79: *Mental retardation*

F80-F89: *Disorders of psychological development*
Here the disorder includes specific developmental disorders of speech and language.
Specific developmental disorders of scholastic skills, specific development disorder of motor function.
Mixed specific developemental disorders, pervasive developmental disorders.

F90-F98: *Behavioral and emotional disorders with onset usually occurring in childhood and adolescence.*
Condition included here are hyperkinetic disorders, conduct disorders, mixed disorders of conduct and emotions, emotional disorders with onset specific to childhood, disorders of social functioning with onset specific to childhood and adolescence, tic disorders.

F99: *Unspecified mental disorder*
It is mental disorder not otherwise specified.
Recently, there has been upsurge interest in multiaxial system to get more complete disgnosis. In this system patients are diagnosed on many separate axes.

REFERENCE

1. US Department of Health and Human Services: Mental health: A report of the surgeon general, Rockville, Md, National Institute of mental Health, 1999.

SUGGESTED READINGS

1. Chodoff P: The changing role of dynamic psychotherapy in psychiatric practice, Psychiatric Services 51:1404-07, 2000.
2. Dyer J, McGuinness T: Resilience: analysis of concept, Arch Psychiatr Nurs 1996;10:276.
3. Harris E, Barraclough B: Excess mortality of mental disorder, Br J Psychiatry; 1998;173:11.
4. Jorm A: Public knowledge and beliefs about mental disorders, British J of Psychiatry 2000;177:396-401.
5. Kendler K: Social support: a genetic-epidemiologic analysis, Am J Psychiatry 1997;154:1398.
6. Kessler R et al: Lifetime and 12-month prevalence of DSM-R psychiatric disorders in the United States, Arch Gen Psychiatry 1994;51:8.
7. Monat A, Lazarus R: Stress and coping, New York, 1991, Columbia University Press.
8. Murray C, Lopez A: The global burden of disease: a comprehensive assessment of mortality and disability from disease, injuries, and risk factors in 1990 and projected to 2020, Cambridge, Mass, 1996, Harvard University Press.
9. Neugebauer R: Mind matters: the importance of mental disorders in public health's 21st century mission, Am J public Health 1999;89:1309.
10. Stuart G, Laraia M: Principles and practice of psychiatric nursing, edn. 7th, St louis, 2001, Mosby.
11. Tucker G: Putting DSM-4 in perspective, Am J psychiatry 1998;155:159.
12. Ustun T: The global burden of mental disorders, Am J Public Health 1999;89:1315.

CHAPTER 6

Communication

INTRODUCTION

Virginia Satir states in her book 'people making' "I see communication as a huge umbrella that covers and affects all that goes on between human beings. Once a human being has arrived on this earth, communication is the largest single factor determining what kinds of relationship he makes with others and what happens to him in the world around him. How he manages his survival, how he develops intimacy, how he makes sense, how he connects with his own divinity—all are largely depend on his communication skills"

Nursing is a profession which depends largely on communication. Nurses have contact with various types of people: patients, family members, other health professionals, and many others. It is very essential for a nurse to develop and utilize communication skills.

What is communication? Communication derived from Latin word *communis* denoting, common. Communication is concerned with imparting a common idea or understanding or exchange of meaning.

DEFINITION

Communication is reciprocal exchange of thoughts, ideas opinions, facts, values feeling attitudes, and wishes, etc.

Communication is an act (behavior) and a process, communicate is a behavior since it always involves physical and mental activity on the part of the sender and receiver of the message. Communication is also a process through which ideas are exchanged. So, in order to communicate there must be a sender (source, encoder) a recipient (receiver) and the meanings (or message) must be understood by the individuals involved.

A circular mode of communication.

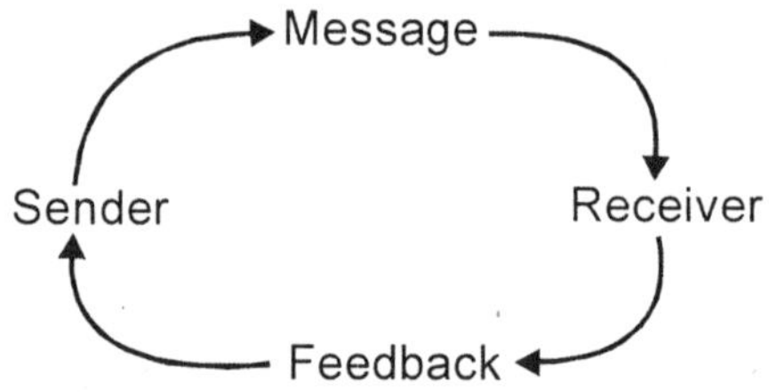

COMMUNICATION MODEL

Communication model compared of six elements (below S.M. C.R model).

1. Referent
2. Source encoder
3. Message
4. Channels
5. Receiver or decoder
6. Feedback

Referent

It is an idea, it may be an object, act, situation or experience, which prompts the source encoder to initiate the communication.

Source Encoder

This is a person who initiates the conversation, and talks about the idea. How much his communication will be effective, depends upon his communication skills, his knowledge about the idea, his attitudes and his sociocultural factors which are always challenging.

The idea expressed by the encoder may not be understood by the decoder if the encoder do not have the ability to encode. The vocal mechanisms used in speech, the motor skills used in writing and the language peculiar to a specific culture are the encoding skills of the encoder. Gestures and non-verbal behaviors are different to different cultures which affects the communication.

Message

It is the content selecting and arrangement of the content is very important in communication.

Channels

These are routs of conveying the message. Channels involve the senses of hearing, seeing, touching, smelling and tasting. The sensory channel selected must be appropriate to the message and should be suitable for the decoder.

Receiver or Decoder

He is the person whom the message is directed. He is also influenced by the same factors of communication, knowledge, attitude and socio-cultural factors.

Feedback

It is the result of the communication. It helps to determine the success or failure of the communication.

LEVEL OF COMMUNICATION

Communication takes place on at least three different levels.
- Intrapersonal
- Interpersonal
- Public communication.

Intrapersonal

This level of communication is what occurs when people communicate within themselves. When a nurse sees a patient pertinent having a wound, thinks "I would better get the wound dressed and give medication". The nurse is communicating intrapersonally.

Interpersonal

This process is primary to other two levels because it involves perception of self and others, it is necessary and important in all communication encounters which takes place between dyads (groups of two persons) and in small groups.

Public Communication

It is communication between a person and several other people. Its most common term is the presentation of a public speech. Mass media is another form of public communication.

TYPES OF COMMUNICATION

There are two types of communication.

Verbal Communication

It occurs through the medium of words, both spoken or written. It can convey factual information accurately and efficiently.

Nonverbal Communication

Non-verbal communication includes everything that does not involve the spoken or written word including all of the five senses. It is said that only 7 percent of meaning is conveyed by words, 35 percent is by paralinguistic cues such as voice and 55 percent is transmitted by body cues. (Suart K Sundeen) More honest messages are communicated by nonverbal communication. It is very important on the part of nurses to develop skills in understanding, nonverbal communication which carry more social meaning than verbal channels.

There is a wide varieties of nonverbal communication like:

- Facial expression
- Hand gestures
- Body movement
- Pitch rate and volume of voice
- Touch
- Body aromas.

These can be discussed in various categories.

Kinesics

The study of body movement as a form of nonverbal communication is called kinesics. Facial expressions, gestures and eye movement are mostly used here.

Facial Expression

Facial expression can convey varies feelings like anger, sad, anxiety, depression, happiness, etc.

Sign Language

Hand gestures can communicate anxiety, indifference and impatience. Foot shuffling and fidgeting may express the desire to exit. Body position give, cues about how open a person is to another person. Feeling of relaxation on stiffness can convey various meaning.

Eye contact is another important cue in communication. It can convey friendly feeling, guilt feeling, love feeling believable and earnest, etc.

Paralanguage

Paralanguage refers to something beyond the language tests.

It has two components.
- Voice quality such as pitch and range
- Nonlanguage vocalization such as sobbing, laughing or grunting (noises without linguistic structure)

These vocal cues can differentiate emotions.

Proximics

Proximics is the study of space relationship maintained by persons in the interaction. How close the person sits with another person gives clue in his behavior.

Touch

Touching behaviors are very much important in communication. Touching can convey many meaning like, support, love, anger, etc.

Cultural Artifacts

Artifacts are items in contact with interacting persons that may act as nonverbal stimuli. Clothes, cosmetics, perfumes, deodorants, jewellery, eye glasses, wigs, and hair pieces, beards and moustaches and so on.

All types of nonverbal messages are important. But interpreting them correctly is essential. The nurse should refer to the specific behavior observed and attempt to confirm its meaning and significance with the patient. If the nurse's words and tone of voice indicate that he or she is truly clarifying, suggesting or validating, a defensive reaction usually is not evoked.

FACTORS THAT INFLUENCE COMMUNICATION

Communication can be effective or ineffective depending upon the following factors:

1. The perception, thought and feelings of the sender and receiver, prior to message transmission. This depends upon to the previous background, attitude towards message, the receiver and her health, etc.
2. The relationship between the sender and the receiver.
3. Intentions of the sender.
4. Content of the message language used arrangement of words and clarity, etc.
5. The context in which the communication taken place, e.g. physical environment and psychological factors related to readiness and timings, etc.
6. Manner in which the message is transmitted, verbal or nonverbal, channels used, etc.
7. Effects of the message the receiver.
8. Cultural context of the sender and receiver.

Though communication is necessary and important always in all walks of life, it has different meaning and utility in psychiatric nursing. The assessment, analysis, diagnosis treatment and rehabilitation of patients with behavioral problems depend upon the effective communication of team members with patient and with in the group. Some of the effecting therapeutic techniques used in psychiatric nursing are discussed in the following pages:

THERAPEUTIC COMMUNICATION TECHNIQUES

There are many communication techniques. Some are therapeutic and some are nontherapeutic. Nurses should be aware of therapeutic techniques of communication and use them in day-to-day conversation with the client. Communication to be most therapeutic. It must convey a respectful attitude, one that supports the individuals and self-esteem of both clients and the nurses. The following are the identified as therapeutic communication technique that allow one to learn how to convey such attitude.

Using Silence

Utilizing absence of verbal command.

Silence often encourages the patient to verbalize if it is an interested expectant silence. This kind of silence indicates to the patient that the nurse expects him to speak to later organize his thoughts, and communication. A positive and accepting silence can be a valuable therapeutic tool.

Acceptance

Giving indication of reception. For example,
" *yes*"
"*uh humm*"
 "*I follow that you said*"
" *Nodding*"
The accepting response indicates that nurse has heard and has followed the trend of patient thought. It also shows nurse is attentive and a participant, not a passive observer. Accepting does not indicate agreement but is non-judgment in character. "It is simply a verbalization of the attitude of permissiveness and acceptance of the nurse which says that you need not be ashamed of expressing how you really feel."

Not only the accepting words are important, but also the facial expression, the tone of voice and posture of the nurse all must convey the same feeling of acceptance.

Giving Recognition: Acknowledging, Indicating Awareness

For example *Goodmorning Mr. S; "I noticed that you have combed your hair..."*

It indicate that nurse recognizes the patient as a person, as an individual.

Offering self

Making one's self-available, for example

I will stay with you'.

I am interested in your welfare'.

I will sit with you for sometime'.

Patient may not be ready to talk to the nurse but the nurse can offer her presence, her interest and her desire to understand. To be therapeutic her offer should be made unconditional that is patient need not be forced or felt that he has to convey his feeling because nurse is offering herself.

Giving Broad Opening

Allowing the patient to take the initiative in starting the conversation.

For example, *Is there something you would like to talk about?*

- *What are you thinking about?*
- *Where would you like to begin?*

Broad opening gives the idea that the lead is to be taken by the patient. It stimulates the patient to take the initiative and to feel that this is what is expected of him. It provides the chance for the patient to ventilate his feelings or allows the patient to talk about his thoughts of the day.

Offering General Leads: In Giving Encouragement to Continue

For example, *"Go on*
　　And then
　　Tell me about it".

　　General leads such as that 'And after that' or 'go on' leave the direction of the discussion entirely on the patient. It indicates that nurse is following what patient is telling and she is interested in what is to come next. Here the verbal activities of the nurse is at a minimum and the patient does most of the talking. The nurse encourages by her nonverbal activities such as nodding or various gestures if verbal activities is necessary she may use one word such as well or really, etc.

Placing the Event in Time or in the Sequence

For example, *" Was this before the incident or after"*.
" When did this happen"?

　　Putting events in their sequence helps both nurse and the patient to see them in perspective. It may help to identify cause-and-effect relationship or a recurrent pattern of interpersonal difficulties.

Making Observation—Verbalizing what is Perceived?

"You appear tense"
"I notice you are restless today".

　　Whatever the observation nurse makes on the patient she should bring, to the awareness of the patient and encourage mutual understanding of the behavior or feeling through discussion. Making observation also indicates that nurse is interested in patient.

Restating—Repeating the Main Idea

For example, *I cannot sleep I stay awake all night.*
Nurse: You have difficulty in sleeping.

Restating is a technique whereby the nurse repeats the main message the patient expressed.

It helps the nurse to verify understanding the patient message and also encourages the patient to continue as he feels that nurse is truly listening and making every attempt to understand him.

Reflecting: Directing back the Patient's Questions, Feeling and Ideas

For example, *patient—My husband spends all my money and then asks me to get more from my parents.*
Nurse—It sounds you are angry on your husband.

Reflection is as its name implies reflecting or interpreting back to the patient what has been heard and understood. It may be a statement such as "it sounds like you are sad, etc.

Reflection is a powerful tool which encourages the patient to bring about his feeling of which the client has not expressed verbally.

Focusing ...... Concentrating on a Single Point

For example *"Let us talk some more about....."*
" *The point seems worth looking at more closely"*.

Focusing is a technique in which the nurse directs the conversation to focus on a topic of particular importance or relevance to the patient. The purpose is to draw the patient attention to the theme—its meaning and significance in patient life and adjustment.

Exploring ... Dealing Further into a Subject or Idea

For example *"Tell me more about that"*
   "Describe it in detail"
   " what kind of job you are doing"?

Exploring more fully certain ideas or experiences of patient are very necessary in therapeutic relationship. Many patients talk very superficially about the important issues. Nurse has to identify the problem and should recognize when to evaluate further. She should not probe, if patient is not willing to elaborate. The nurse should respect the patient wishes.

Giving Information

For example *"Visiting hours are"*
"At this time you are expected to do"....

Giving information is providing necessary facts and information to the patient. It may be about his illness, the etiology, treatment, prognosis, legal aspects of case or rules and regulation of hospital, etc. Giving information builds up trust, as well as gives the patient a greater body of knowledge from which to make decisions. Here nurse acts as a resource person.

Seeking Clarification...

Seeking to make clear which is not meaningful or vague. For example *"Are you saying that"*
"I am not sure what you mean. Could you tell me that again"?

Clarification or a technique where the nurse tries to put the patient ideas into a simple statement. She might say " Are you saying that " .. and till the manages, she has heard to check her understanding and to make the patient's thoughts or feelings explicit. This also indicates the genuine interest of nurse on the patient.

Presenting Reality

Offering in consideration that which is real.

For example *"I see no one else in the room"*.
"For me your mother seems to be good and caring".

When it is obvious that the patient is misinterpreting reality, the nurse can indicate that which is real. This should not be like arguing with the patient or belittling his own experience, but tells rather by calmly and quickly expressing her own perceptions. The intention here is merely to indicate an alternate line of thought in the patient to consider, not to 'convince' that he is wrong.

Voicing Doubt

Expressing uncertainties or doubting the patient's perception.
For example, *Isn't that unusual?*
It's Really?
That's hard to believe.

Another means of responding to distortions of reality is to express doubt. Such expression permits patient to become aware that others do not necessarily perceive what he perceives and this gives an idea to reconsider or re-evaluate what has occurred.

Seeking Consensual Validation

Searching in mutual understanding for accord in the meaning of words.
For example, *"Tell me whether my understanding of it agrees with yours"*.
"Are you conveying the idea that..."?

Some words give different meaning to different people. So when it is doubtful the nurse has to suggest" "Are you using this phrase to convey the idea ..."?

Recognizing and Reflecting the Feeling (Verbal or nonverbal)

Voicing what the patient has hinted or seeing to verbalize the feeling that are being expressional indirectly.
For example, *Verbal-patient—I can't talk to you or to anyone. It's waste of time. Non-verbal—Is it your feeling, that no one understand you.*

Patient — I am dead.

Nurse: Are you suggesting that you feel lifeless?

Summarizing

Organizing and summing up that has gone before.
For example, *"During the past hour you and I have discussed".*
"You have said that ....."

Summarization brings together the important points of the discussion and gives each participant an awareness of the progress made. It allows both nurse and patient to depart with the same ideas in mind and provides a sense of closure at the completion of each discussion.

Encouraging Formulation of a Plan of Action

Asking the patient to consider kinds of behavior likely to be appreciated in future situation.
"What you will do to let your anger, without harming others?
"How you will handle the situation next time"?

This will be helpful for the patient to plan for the future to handle various interpersonal crisis situations.

Nurse may encourage the patient to talk it out the plan of action and guide in planning and executing. She may encourage the patient roleplay or act out with her such situation in advance as another means of preparation.

In a broad score, the entire nurse-patient relationship is an experience of this sort 'a preview of future relationships of a mere reciprocal nature in which the patient may find and give-acceptance, respect and understanding.

NONTHERAPEUTIC TECHNIQUES

False Reassuring

Indicating that there is no cause for anxiety.
For example, *Everything will be all right.*
" *Don't worry about it".*
" *you are doing fine".*

Telling that there is no sufficient reason for patient's anxiety to be brought down.

Indicates devaluating patient's own feeling.

Hence, no value is placed on patient's judgment.

The nurse communicates only her lack of understanding and empathy. If it is a patient's progress she wants to comment upon, she can offer concrete examples of changes that have excused rather than starting "you are doing fine".

Buston tells us that giving reassurance is a common error, it makes the person giving it feel better in a short-time but is meaningless to the patient in longer duration.

Refusing

Refusing to consider or showing contemplation for the patient idea or behavior.
For example, *"Let us not discuss"*
"I don't want to hear about".

When any topic is rejected, it is closed off from explanation. When the patient himself is rejected, therapeutic interaction ceases. It is said that insecure therapist is likely to be afraid of the patient anxiety producing experience.

Disapproving

Denouncing the patient's behavior or ideas
For example, *"That's bad"*.
"I' d rather you could not".

Disapproval implies that the nurse has the right to pay judgment on the patent's thought and actions.

It further implies that the patient is expected to please the Nurse. Nurse is supported to accept the patient as he is being neither moralistic nor conditional.

Advising

Telling the patient what to do.
For example *"I think you should"*.
"Why don't you".

When the nurse tell the patient what he should do and it implies that the nurse knows what is best for him so the patient is incapable of any self-direction.
Paplau States that advice acts to prevent the patient from struggling with and thinking through her problems.

Probing

Persistent questioning of the patient.
For example *"Now tell me about"*.
"Tell me your life history".

Probing makes the patient determine. He may respond with anger, with distortions or cease to respond entirely.

Challenging

Demanding proof from the patient.
For example, *"How can you be the president of India"?*
"If you are dead, why is your heart beating"?

Often the nurse feels that if she challenges the patient to prove his unrealistic ideas, he will realize that he has no "proof" and will be tried to acknowledge what is "true" she forgets the delusional ideas serve a purpose and not given up so readily when challenged, the patient tends become.

Introducing an Unrelated Topic

Changing the subject
For example, *Patient: I would like to die.*
Nurse: Did you have visitors the weekend?

When the nurses changes the subject or introduces one, she takes over the direction of the discussion. This can be done only when there are delusional ideas expressed by the patient otherwise she has to listen to the thoughts and feeling of the patient which will help the patient to understand better.

Using the therapeutic techniques the nurse does the 'process recording' which is one important activity of a psychiatric nurse throughout the stay of the patient with her. The following chapters discusses the process recording in detail.

CHAPTER 7

Therapeutic Nurse-Patient Relationship

INTRODUCTION

There are various kinds of relationships, social relationship, personal relationship, friendly relationship, etc. But the nurse-patient relationship is therapeutic relationship, which is professional one.

Sullian and few others have suggested the cause of mental illness may be faulty interpersonal relationship at different developmental stages. So, the treatment of mental illness has to be based on strong supportive and helping interpersonal relationship.

The therapeutic nurse patient-relationship is a mutual learning experience and a corrective emotional experience for the patient. Here the nurse uses self and clinical techniques in working with the patient to bring about insight and behavioral changes in the patient.

The Goals of Nurse-Patient Relationship

The goals of nurse-patient relationship are:
1. Patient develops self realization, self acceptance and increased self respect.
2. Patient develops clear sense of personal identity and personal integration.

3. Develops ability to form intimate interdependent, interpersonal relationship.
4. Has improved functioning.
5. And achieves realistic personal goals.

To achieve the above goals, good nurse-patient relationship is very important, where nurse explores various experiences of the patient, make the patient to express his thoughts, perceptions and feelings. Areas of conflicts and anxieties are identified and clarified. Problems of communication are corrected, maladaptive behavior pattern are modified and more adaptive coping mechanisms are learnt.

'Self-understanding' and 'communication techniques' are the tools used in psychiatric nursing.

THERAPEUTIC USE OF SELF

Self analysis is an essential aspect of therapeutic nursing care. She must have:
1. Self awareness.
2. Clarifies her own values now and then.
3. Explores her own feelings towards patient and his problems.
4. Serve as role model.
5. Has altruistic motivation.
6. Follows sense of ethics and responsibility.

PHASES OF RELATIONSHIP

1. Hildegard E Paplau (1952) identifies four phases in the relationship. They are: orientation, identification, exploration, and resolution. Each phase characterized by overlapping roles or function in relation to health problem as nurse and patient learn to work cooperatively to resolve difficulties.

2. Staurt (2002) and others talks about four phases in nurse-patient relationship.
   a. Preorientation phase
   b. The orientation phase or introductory phase
   c. Working phase
   d. The termination phase.

The Preorientation or Preinteraction Phase

The preinteraction phase involves preparation of the nurse for the first time meeting with the client.

1. Here the nurse gets available information about the patient from the casefile, significant others or from other team members.
2. She examines her own feelings, fears, anxieties about the patient's history, diagnosis, etc. For example, nurse may be having an ambivalent feeling towards alcoholic patients because of her past personal experience. She should be aware of her feelings and preconception that may affect her interpersonal relationship. She analysis her own professional strength weakness and limitations.
3. She plans for the first meet with the patient.

Orientation Phase

In orientation phase the nurse meets the patient first time, introduces herself and determines why the patient sought help.

The tasks included here are:

1. Nurse creates an environment for establishment of trusting relationship.
2. Establishes a contract for interaction including the expectations and responsibilities of nurse and patient.
3. Gathers assessment information to build a strong patient database.

4. Explores patients thought, feelings and actions.
5. Identify patient problems, strength or limitations.
6. Formulates nursing diagnosis.
7. Set goals that are mutually agreeable to the nurse and patient.
8. Develops a plan of action that is realistic for meeting the goal.
9. Explores the feelings of both the patient and nurse interims of the introductory phase.

During introductory phase both nurse and patient may have some anxiety. Until a degree of rapport has been established.

Working Phase

Most of the therapeutic work is carried out during the working phase. Here the tasks included are:
1. Maintaining the trust and rapport that was established.
2. The nurse and the patient explore relevant stressors and promote the development of insight in the patient and perception of reality.
3. Solve the patient problem.
4. Overcome the resistance behavior on the parts of the patient as the level of anxiety rises in response to the discussions.
5. Continuously evaluate the progress toward goal attainment.

Termination Phase

There are various reasons for termination of the phase. They may be:
1. The mutually agreed goals may have been reached.
2. The patient may be discharged from the hospital.

Termination is one of the most difficult but important phases of therapeutic nurse-patient relationship. Here the learning is maximized for patient and nurse. It is time to exchange feelings and memories and to evaluate mutually the patients progress and goal attainments.

The tasks included are:

1. Establish reality of separation.
2. Review progress has been made towards the attainment of goal.
3. Recognize and explore the feelings of termination of relationship, like feelings of rejection, loss, sadness, anger, etc. Both the nurse and patient may experience feelings of sadness and loss, etc. The nurse should share her feelings with the patient. Because the patient learns that it is acceptable to undergo these feelings.
4. A plan for continuing care or for assistance during stressful life experiences is mutually established.

In order to reduce the tension of termination like feelings of rejection, sadness, anger, etc. and to make the termination healthy and easy it is important that the preparation for termination starts at the stage of orientation. When the nurse introduces herself to the patient at the orientation phase, says how long she is going to be working with the patient. As the time of termination is approaching, she will be reminding him how many more days they will be working together. Patient is made gradually independent. This will avoid problems in termination phase.

The phases of the nurse-patient relationship follow the steps of the nursing process.

The orientation phase is assessment phase. The time of getting to know each other and gathering information.

The working phase begins with establishing goals and setting plans for nursing care.

The termination phase comes about during evaluation when it becomes clear that the goals are met and patient is ready to stop the relationship.

Relationship of the Nursing Process with Phases of the Nurse-Patient Relationship

Steps of Nursing Process	Phases of the Nurse-Patient Relationship
Assessment	Orientation phase
identification, diagnosis/ planning/intervention	Working phase
Evaluation	Termination phase

QUALITIES AND SKILLS NECESSARY FOR THERAPEUTIC RELATIONSHIP

The nurse must acquire certain skills or qualities to initiate and continue a therapeutic relationship. They are broadly divided into responsive and action dimension.

RESPONSIVE DIMENSIONS

Genuineness

Genuineness refers to the ability to be real or honest with another. It is closely related to the respect dimension because 'we are most genuine with those for whom we care most.' Artificiality, even with a purpose of adopting a scientific principle will interfere with a relationship. If the patient recognizes that the nurse is not genuine (sincere) he may loose confidence in her. Genuineness implies that the nurse is an open person who is self-congruent, authentic and accessible.

Respect

Patient is an individual with his own values, interests, believes and opinion. Nurse has to respect him as a person.

The respect can be conveyed by:
- Listening to the patient
- Encouraging to put forward his plans of actions
- Being honest with him
- Giving privacy whenever needed.

Empathic Understanding

Putting oneself in the shoes of another" is a way of describing empathy. It is defined as "an ability to feel with the patient while retaining an ability to critically analyze the situation". Empathy is an important dimension in the helping process. It helps in interpersonal exploration.

To be able to empathize the nurse must be willing to get involved enough to feel what the other person feels at the same time avoid over-involvement, projection and over-identification which is harmful. An ability to identify and use imagination is important in the process of empathizing.

Concreteness

Nurse should use specific terminology rather than abstraction while discussing with patient's feelings, experiences and behavior. Whatever she speaks should have clarity.

ACTION ORIENTED DIMENSION

Confrontation

A confrontation is a deliberate invitation to another to examine some aspect of personal behavior in which there is discrepancy between what the person says and what he or she does.

Confrontation requires careful attention to nonverbal communication and the discrepancies between verbal and nonverbal messages.

It will help the patient's self awareness and productive changes occur from constructive confrontations.

The six skills involved in constructive confrontation are:

1. The use of personal statements with the words I, my and me.
2. The use of relationship statements in which the nurse expresses what she thinks or feels about the patient interaction.
3. The use of the behavior description.
4. The use of description of personal feelings.
5. The use of responses aimed at understanding such as para phrasing and perception checking.
6. The use of constructive feedback.

Immediacy

Responding with immediacy means responding to what is happening between the nurse and the patient in here and now. Current nurse-patient interaction in relationship is used to learn about patients functioning in other interpersonal relationships.

Emotional Catharsis

Patient is encouraged to talk about most bothering aspects of life, for therapeutic effect.

Good listening and support to be given during catharsis.

Nurse Disclosure

Sometimes the nurse reveals information about self and own ideas, values, feelings and attitudes to facilitate patients cooperation, learning, catharsis or support.

Role Playing

Patient should be encouraged to act out a particular situation when he is having problem. It will help to increase patients' insight into human relations. Patient to see a situation from another point of view. It will allow the patient to experiment with new behavior in a safe environment.

The action dimensions must be implemented in the context of warmth, acceptance and understanding established by the responsive dimension. They will help in therapeutic relationship by identifying obstacles, which interferes patient growth and help in self awareness and behavioral change.

THERAPEUTIC IMPASSES

There are few obstacles, which can occur, in therapeutic nurse-patient relationships. They are:
1. Resistance.
2. Transference.
3. Counter transference.
4. Boundary violation.

They arise due to various reasons. Some may be due to clients' pathology, or lack of knowledge. Some may be due to nurses' own inability to be effective due to inexperiences, lack of knowledge or personal problems. They all stall the therapeutic relationship. Nurse has to deal with them as soon as it occurs. These reactions can produce intense feelings to the client and the nurse.

Resistance

Resistance occurs when the patient consciously or unconsciously conceals the problems even the signs and symptoms. This may be to avoid anxiety. This is a natural reluctance or learned avoidance of verbalizing or experiencing the troubled aspect of oneself. A primary resistance is often the patience unwillingness to change, when a need for change is recognized.

Forms of resistance displayed by the patients are:
- Suppression and repression of pertinent information
- Intensification of symptoms
- Acting out
- Superficial talk
- Intellectual inhibitions like breaking appointments be forgetful, be silent, sleepy during session
- Having transference reaction, etc.

When resistance occurs, it must be addressed and dealt with by both nurse and the client. Nurses can help client to overcome resistance by pointing out their progress and strength, which can lessen the anxiety.

Transference

Transference is an unconscious response whereby client identifies the nurse with some one significant to their life. Feelings and attitudes about the other person are transferred to the nurse. For example, A patient can see the nurse as a mother figure, because she has a similar mannerism to his own mother. She may have negative feeling about his mother. So, without provocation she becomes angry on the nurse. Transference reactions are harmful to the therapeutic processes if they are ignored and unexamined by the nurse.

Nurse should deal with transference by being prepared to hear the client's rational and highly charged emotions. She must listen patiently using the communicative techniques of clarifying and reflecting to begin problem solving.

The final goal is the client gain awareness of his problem and recognizes the reason for his resistance.

Counter Transference

This is a therapeutic impass created by the nurse. Here the nurse identifies the patient with someone significant to her life. This emotional response by the nurse to the patient is inappropriate to the content and context of therapeutic relationship.

Counter transference reactions are usually of three types:

1. Reactions of intense love or caring.
2. Reactions of intense anxiety.
3. Reaction of hostility.

Forms of counter transference displayed by nurses:

- Difficulty in empathizing with the patient
- Feeling angry or impatient during the session
- Feeling depressed after session/drowsy during session
- Encouraging patients dependency/praise
- Personal or social involvement
- Dreaming about the patient
- Coming late to the session or running overtime
- Arguing with the patient, etc.

To deal with counter transference the nurse must conduct an honest self-appraisal throughout the therapeutic relationship. If the self-appraisal reveals any problem, she must explore why it is occurring. If she cannot handle alone, she should get some help from professionals to deal with it.

Boundary Violations

Boundary violation occur when a nurse goes beyond the established therapeutic relationship and enters into a social, economic or personal relationship with patient.

Possible boundary violation related to psychiatric nurses

- Patient takes the nurse out for lunch or dinner
- Nurse attends a party along with the patient or with patients invitation
- Nurse accepts gifts from the patient
- Professional relationship turns into personal relationship
- Nurse does business with the patient
- Nurse very often talks about her personal matters with patient
- Nurse meets the patient for treatment outside hospital settings.

OVERCOMING THERAPEUTIC IMPASSES

1. The nurse should be prepared to be exposed to powerful emotional feelings.
2. She must have knowledge about the impasses and recognize them at the early stage.
3. She should clarify and reflect on feelings and content to know objectively what is happening.
4. The reason behind the behavior must be explored.
   - For resistance and transference patient should be made to understand the reason behind the problem and deal with it.
5. For counter transference and boundary violations the nurse accept the responsibility and try to solve

the problem either on her own or by some other's help.

6. The goal of the relationship and patient needs and problems to be reviewed.

7. Re-establish therapeutic relationship to achieve the identified goal.

Establishing nurse-patients relationship is a major skill necessary to provide care to psychiatric patients. The therapeutic, professional relationships is always necessary for assessment, setting up realistic goal, to work towards the goal and to make the patients more independent in solving his own problems.

CHAPTER 8

Process Recording and Nursing Care Plan

INTRODUCTION

Process Recording

Recording or documentation is an important and necessary function of any organization. Whether it is an industry, business, hospital or even farming. Till the time of Florence Nightingale it is not considered that documentation is necessary for the work nurses do. Since the time of Florence Nightingale nurses have viewed documentation as a necessary action. During this time documentation was primarily a mean to communicate, implement the medical orders, not for observation or assessment of the patient's status. So, the nursing documentation never found a place in the case files of patients after discharge.

In early 1970's due to the changes in nursing practice, establishment of regulatory agencies and legal guidelines, nursing documentation has become more important in patient care.

Documentation is necessary because of many reasons. They are:

Accountability

The individual who is employed has the accountability to the employer directly, though the work he is entrusted. He does the work not only by doing but by recording also.

Legal Protection

In every field either it is in the business or in hospital people are aware of their rights. Human right commission is very active to protect the rights of the individual so many action done, for patient's are to be recorded for legal purpose.

Helps in Evaluation or Outcome of Nursing Care

Nursing care has different steps and evaluation in the last but important step. Process recording is an evaluation tool in psychiatric nursing.

It is a Record to Communicate to the Colleagues

Handing over and taking over is done orally but process recording will be the written, record for the colleagues to refer.

It also helps to Communicate to Other Team Members

Any team member at anytime can refer these process recording for the clarification, diagnosis and treatment. Documentation or recording is done in different ways in different situations. Process recording is a method of recording used in psychiatric wards by nurses.

PROCESS RECORDING

Definition

"The recording of the conversation during the interaction or the interview between the nurse and the

patient in the psychiatric setup, with nurses inference is called process recording."

This will help the nurses to know the patients better so that the nurse can evaluate the patient.

It is used as an:

- Evaluation tool
- Diagnostic tool
- Teaching tool/ Educative
- Therapeutic tool
- Prerequisition for nursing process.

Evaluation Tool

The consequent process recording from the day I and later will help the nurses and the team members to know the patient and also the change in the behavior with the treatment given. This can be used in the practical examination by which the examiner can evaluate the student whether she understood the mental mechanisms that patient was using and also the student can do the inference and here the examiner can also test the ability of the student to use the different communication techniques.

Diagnostic Tool

Histories given by the patient or family members may not sufficient or correct to do the diagnosis. But the record of the verbatim of the patient during the next interview may reveal more information. This will help to confirm the diagnosis or to change the diagnosis.

Teaching/Education

The senior nurses and the teachers use these techniques to teach the student and junior nurses.

Therapeutic Tool

The nurse use this opportunity to guide the patient, suggest and correct the behavior after the introducing sessions.

Process recording in Psychiatric nursing has many advantages. They are:
1. It helps the nurse to keep rapport with the patient
2. To know the symptoms of the patient
3. To know the psychodynamics of the patient
4. To plan the short-term goals of nursing care
5. To plan the long-term goals of nursing care
6. To prepare the patient and family for rehabilitation and follow-up.

TIME LIMIT

The total time spent for recording should be 30 minutes. The active phase can be 20 minutes with 10 minutes for conclusion and recording.

PRE-REQUISITE FOR PROCESS RECORDING

1. Consent from the patient if the patient is oriented to time, place, and person
2. Set the objective for each session.

The objectives of process recording are important responsibilities of the nurse. These objectives are set according to the day of the admission of the patient and also according to the condition of the patient.

Common objectives in different stages are given below.

During Acute Stage

- To establish rapport with patient
- To know the psychotic ideas

- To divert the patient from destructive activities
- To keep him engaged.

During First Meeting with a Patient

- Does not have any acute disturbing symptoms.
- To explore the personal history.
- To identify any psychotic ideas (Hallucination/illusion).
- To establish rapport.
- To improve interpersonal relationship.
- To know the hobbies and interest so that planning can be done when get discharged.

WHEN SYMPTOMS ARE ABSENT/GETTING READY FOR DISCHARGE

- To plan for discharge.
- To improve the family role or involvement.
- To emphasize the need for long-term treatment.
- To make him understand the need for regular follow-up.
- To give knowledge of early symptoms of drug toxicity, etc.

FORMAT FOR PROCESS RECORDING

Identification of the patient
- Personal histories
  - Birth
  - Milestones
  - Scholastic performance
  - Peer interaction
  - Employment
  - Marital history
- Socioeconomic status

- Family histories of
  - Father—age, education, employment, communication
  - Mother
  - Siblings
  - Spouse and children.
- Medical histories—Past/Present
- Present existing complaints
- Provisional diagnosis
- Objectives.

VERBATIM 1

Exact: Place

Date and time –

Situation –

On which day of admission –

Table. 8.1: Person verbatim nonverbal communication inference techniques used by the nurse are included in process recording

Person	Verbatam	Nonverbal communication	Communication inference technique used by the nurse
Nurse			
patient			

At the end of the conversation nurse should write any special difficulties faced during the interview.Time and place of next interview also can be given to patient and nursing care plan can be included.

Signature

Conclusion: Fixing the time and place for the next interview.

Summary: List of inferences

Care Plans: According to the inferences.

NURSING CARE PLAN

Nursing care plans are written document of what nurses do for the patients for their specific problems. The permanent record of such plans can be considered as part.

Medical Legal Record

Standard guidelines are used while planning for nursing action. But specific plans are executed according to the needs of individual patients. Through the planned nursing care, the nurse demonstrates her nursing skills, her scientific knowledge, her psychological and sociological insight into the problems of the patients and her skill in interpersonal relations with the patients and the family members.

DEFINITION

It is a plan of action which includes a resume of the patient's problems, a nursing diagnose based on observation a description of the proposed nursing approach and a continuous evaluation of the effectiveness of the nursing action.

Different steps in nursing can plan:

1. Gather the information.
   a. Study the medical history and clinical records.
   b. Interview the patient.
   c. Observe the patient continuously.
2. Analyses the information
   a. Evaluate the collected data review the history, physician records, information from family members
   b. List the problems according to the priority
   c. Develop nursing interventions or action by:

      i.   Stating the goals

      ii.   Identifying the problems

      iii. Making the nursing diagnoses

      iv. Explain the patient his/her level of under-standing

      v.   Keep the plans flexible to meet the patients changing needs.

d. Evaluate the effectiveness of the nursing action and modify the action if needed to attain the goal.

The goal can be again divided into two groups according to the priority which are referred as short-terms goals and long-term goods. The short-terms goals are the goals which aim at immediate relief of symptoms like violence, lack of personnel hygiene, food refusal, etc. but long-term goal are aimed at complete freedom from symptoms correcting the family pathology, plan for rehabilitation, helping for drug complaining, placement, etc.

In conclusion the nursing care plan is valid and practiced throughout the hospital stay of the patient with different goals on different day of admission it can be in 16.11 's , crisis intervention, progressive patients care.

NURSING CARE PLAN: IT CAN BE USED AS

- Part of nursing
- To teach the students
- To evaluate the students
- To evaluate our own knowledge and skills
- To evaluate and to be evaluated by the peer groups.

Performa Used in Nursing Care Plan

The nursing care plan is written either along with the care study or without case study.

If it is with care study use the case study performa. If nursing care plan is written without case study what is usually done by the staff nurses in the word consist of two parts.

Bio-data: Name, age, sex, chief complaints, direction and other medical problem treatment of any; date of admission only once in the beginning.

Short-term goals : Long-terms goals.

Nursing care plan is written in different columns.

Table 8.2: Nursing care plan

Identifi-cation of problems	Nursing diagnosis	Nursing interventions /actions	Rationale	Evaluation

1. *Identification of problems* These problems are written in Laymans language, and what the nurses observe on the patient. For example,
   a. Raised body temperate not that patient is having fever.
   b. Looks dirty, not that patient is lacking personnel hygiene.
2. *Nursing diagnosis* This time the nurse can use the NANDA classification of nursing diagnose which is given in the book Chapter 5.
3. *Intervention/action* This is done according to symptoms and the severety of the symptoms. In other words, the nurse has to see the priority and do accordingly.

4. *Rationale* Here the nurse has to mention how their action relives the symptoms.
5. *Evaluation* Evaluation can be done objectively, subjectively and even by the peer group or other team members.

If the patient is with family members or community agencies the nurse can teach them or explains them the scientific reasons of her intervention during the patients stay in the hospital. So, that they can use these techniques or action after the discharge. Other procedure like nursing process and process recording also interlinked with nursing care plan but basic action nursing care plan.

BIBLIOGRAPHY

1. Abrham Varghese: An introduction to psychiatric the Christian Literature Society–Madras, 1976.
2. Bimla Kapoor: Textbook of Psychiatric Nursing kumar publisher Delhi, 1994.
3. Mary Verghese: Essential of Psychiatric and Mental Health Nursing. BI Churchill Livingstone Pvt. Ltd. New Delhi, 1994.

CHAPTER 9

Treatment Modalities Used for Maladaptive Behaviors

INTRODUCTION

There are various kinds of treatment modalities used to cure the mentally ill from time to time. Though no specific treatment had been so far identified as sure cure for any mental illness, a combination of various kinds of treatment has been used to treat the mental illness.

Before the development of scientific theories for the cause of mental illness, people were using starvation, purging, ice-cold packs, burning, keeping the patient in temple, etc. After invention of drugs, the mode of treatment is changed tremendously. At present there are various kinds of treatment like physical, psychological, social, occupational and other therapies used to treat the mentally ill.

METHODS OF TREATMENT

The treatment methods discussed in this chapter are:
1. Pharmacotherapies
2. Physical Therapies
   - Electroconvulsive Therapy (ECT)
   - Phototherapy
3. Psychotherapy

- Individual therapy
- Group therapy
- Family therapy
- Marital therapy
4. Social Therapy
   - Milieu therapy
   - Activity therapy
   - Art therapy
   - Recreation therapy
   - Dance therapy
   - Music therapy
   - Psychodrama
5. Complementary Therapy
   - Relaxation
   - Hypnotherapy
   - Massage and touch
   - Pet assisted therapy.

Pharmacotherapy

The invention of psychotherapeutic drugs has enacted a major change in the management of patient. The drugs are very effective in controlling the symptoms and return the patient to the community and most of the time helps the patient to treat in the community without admitting to the hospital.

The details of the pharmacotherapy and nurses responsibilities are given in the Chapter 27.

Physical Therapies

Somatic therapies are treatment approaches that use physiological or physical interventions to effect behavior change.

Electroconvulsive Therapy (ECT)

- Electroconvulsive therapy is a type of somatic treatment in which electrodes placed on the temples of the patient.
- It is a therapy in which the clients are treated with pulse of electrical energy sufficient to cause a brief convulsions or seizure.
- ECT is one of the most potent and sometimes lifesaving treatment in psychiatry.

Brief History

Von Meduna in 1934 used 25 percent camphor in oil intramuscularly to produce convulsions for the treatment therapeutic purpose, later used Metrazol for the same purpose.

A safer form of convulsive therapy was given by Cerelelti Bini in, 1983. They called it as EST electroshock therapy later known as ECT. There was widespread criticism of ECT and many legislations passed in US restricting its usage. Following this, modifications were made to make it safer.

The American Psychiatric Association (APA) task free on ECT in 1976 gave a report which provided clear guidelines for use ECT and declared it to be safe and effective method of treatment when used by professional trained in the technology.

Purpose

The objective of ECT is to produce a seizure which is established as the essential ingredient for therapeutic effect.

Fraser (1982) states that the therapeutic effect of ECT is most likely due to an alteration in the post-synaptic response to the neurotransmitters in the central nervous system. ECT stimulates synaptic remodeling, causing an increase in synaptic protein. It is the increased synaptic protein that is thought to enhance positive behavior and result in the relief of symptoms.

Duration of Therapy

The usual dose of electric stimulus given to produce seizure is 90-150 volts (average 110) for 0.1—0.5 second (average 0.6 seconds).

Total duration and number of treatments depends on the diagnosis, presence of side effects and response to treatment. Usually, 6-10 treatments are given occasionally up to 15 treatments.

Mechanism of Action

Exact mechanism is unclear. One hypothesis states that it affects the catecholamine pathways between diencephalon (seizure generation area) and limbic system (which is responsible for mood disorder) and also involve hypothalamus.

Another hypothesis says that it produces biochemical changes in the brain—an increase in the level of nor-epinephrine and serotonin.

Indications of ECT

Depressive illness

- Used as an emergency treatment in highly suicidal clients
- In Elderly, ECT may safer than drugs
- Depressive stupor
- Depression with paranoid delusions

- Severe puerparial depression
- Inability to tolerate side effects of antidepressants
- Inability to take drugs. For example, depression in first trimester of pregnancy
- Depression in physical illness—liver and renal failure.

Schizophrenia

ECT provides greater early symptomatic relief than neuroleptic. When both are given the benefit is maximum.

Mania

ECT produces greater and rapid symptom relief. The main indication is excited or uncooperative behavior.

Postpartum psychosis

Some reports that ECT is the treatment of choice in pureparial psychosis and safer in mothers who are breastfeeding.

Schizo Affective Disorders

Other Conditions

Patient with hypochondriac neurosis may have an underlying depression responds to ECT better.

Contraindications of ECT

1. Patient with raised intracranial pressure
2. History of cerebral infarction, aneurysm
3. Cardiac disease
4. Pulmonary disease (TB Pneumonia, Asthma, etc)

TYPES OF ECT

Direct ECT

ECT is given in the absence of muscular relaxation and general anesthesia. This is not common now.

Modified ECT

ECT is modified by drug-induced muscular relaxation and general anesthesia.

Preparation

- ECT is usually administered in the morning
- Fasting at least for 4 hours is a must
- Oral medication should not be given before ECT
- Bladder should be emptied before the ECT
- Loose teeth should be ruled out
- Denture, metallic and sharp objects are removed
- Patient has to be dressed in loose cloth.

After the above preparations patient is placed on a hard bed which is well-insulated. A slow IV drip is started and Inj. Atropine ful 1 ml (0.6 mg) Im/subcutaneous is given 30 min before the treatment, to decreases oral secretion and to prevent vagal stimulation during ECT which causes cardiac arrest. This is the drug of choice.

At the beginning of ECT IV sodium pentathol antathal (5 mg/ng body weight) is given. After this, the muscle relaxant succynyl choline (1 mg/ng body weight) is given, followed by oxygen.

An airway is inserted. The neck extended and the jaw pulled forward to prevent tongue falling back and obstructing the air passage and also to prevent tongue bite during convulsion. The major joints like knee and shoulder are restrained to prevent dislocation and fracture due to violent contraction during ECT.

'U' shaped electrodes are moistened with electrolyte jelly or 25 percent biocorbonate solution should be applied on each side of the temple.

Bilateral ECT, on each sides of the temple and one side of the temple (non-dominant region) in case of unilateral ECT is given. The interelectrode scalp area should be dry and electrode should be applied firmly throughout the passage of the current. The administrator should have dry hand and avoid direct contact with metallic parts of the electrodes. The usual dosage of electricity to get adequate seizure response is 70 to 150 volts from 0.1 to 0.5 sec. The amount of current passed is 200 to 1600 MA. The therapeutic adequacy of the treatment is gauzed by a generalized tonic clinic seizure lasting for not less than 25 to 30 seconds. If the stimulus has failed to elicit a convulsion or if the convulsion has not been adequate, re-stimulation is done subjected to the action of muscle relaxant.

The patient is re-oxygenated after seizure until he resumes regular and spontaneous respiration. A careful watch is made for prolonged post-treatment apnea.

Side Effect of ECT

- ECT produces side effects like amnesia confusion
- Memory impairment which is reversible
- Palpitation and nausea, vomiting, dizziness, dryness of mouth, headache, weakness, fatigue, muscle pain
- Unsteady gait, poor concentration, drowsiness, anxiety restlessness, sweating, respiratory distress, incontinence.

Complications of ECT

- The mortality rate is very low
- Respiratory arrest can occur due to anesthesia and muscle relaxant

- Occasional back pain for few days
- Fractures
- Cardiac dysrhythmia in aged with history of coronary disease
- Memory loss is a transient side effect.

NURSES ROLE

Before ECT

1. Detailed medical and psychiatric history including current and post-treatment history was to be taken.
2. General and physical examination to be done.
3. See that routine laboratory investigations are done and reports are filled.
4. Examination of fundus to rule out papilledema.
5. An informed consent after explaining the procedure to the significant family members.
6. Remove oil from hair.
7. Replace the long acting sedatives with hypnotics.
8. Nil orally at least 8 hours, before treatment.
9. In case of emergency 3 to 4 hours after meal.
10. Remove metallic articles, artificial dentures, lipstick nail polish.
11. Patient should be dressed up in loose clothes.
12. Bladder should be emptied before ECT.
13. Administer pre-medication as ordered.
14. Take the patient on a stretcher to the waiting room.

DURING ECT

1. Transfer the patient on a trolley in a dorsal position/supine position to ECT room.
2. Anesthetic medicine is to be administered.
3. Well-padded mouthgag or airway is placed.

4. Support the shoulder and arms lightly. Restrain the thigh.
5. Hyperextension of the head with support to the chin to be done.
6. Few breaths of oxygen to the patient given.
7. Provide electrodes dipped in saline water or jelly for placing on the temporal region.
8. Observation of patient for seizure, duration, nature, any others, and record.
9. Suction immediately.
10. Restore respiration by oxygen with mask if required.
11. Detail observation and recording.

After ECT

1. Place the patient on lateral position and put the railings.
2. Transfer the patient to post ECT room when he responds to calls.
3. Observe and record pulse, respiration, BP, and level of consciousness every 15 minutes. Once the vital signs are stabilized, record every 30 minutes till the patient recovers completely.
4. Allow the patient to sleep for about 30 minutes, to 1 hour and again this depends on the condition of the patient.
5. Reassure the patient.
6. Re-orient to the ward.
7. Note any injuries, complain of pain or headache.
8. Allow the patient to take food if there is no vomiting.
9. Allow the patient to carry on his routine.
10. His conversation and behavior has to be recorded in detail.
11. Make observation of any change.

PHOTOTHERAPY OR LIGHT THERAPY

Is a new form of treatment used in the treatment of seasonal affective disorder (SAD), a nonpsychotic depression that occurs repeatedly during the winter months. It is seen in the areas of high latitude where daylight time during winter is limited. The depressive symptoms include increased fatigue, weight gain and carbohydrate craving, etc.

Effects of Light Therapy

Clients with SAD are exposed to bright, artificial 5 to 6 hours per day. Antidepressant effects are observed within 4 to 5 days.

It is given till the outdoor light is sufficient to maintain good mood and high energy.

Role of nurse is assessment of SAD case finding and referral to SAD treatment.

Psychotherapy

Psychotherapy is the treatment of mental or emotional disorders. Through psychological rather than physical methods. It is often done in conjunction with somatic therapies, especially medications.

Psychotherapy can be done with individuals or with groups.

Individual Psychotherapy

Use of psychological technique applied in a one-to-one setting. These techniques are designed to help persons overcome mental distress and illness for the purpose of assisting the individuals to reach their optimum level of health. The effectiveness of such therapy depends on the patient therapist relationship.

There are multiple approaches to therapy.

Insight Oriented Therapy

It derives from psychoanalysis for helping the individual to gain insight into feelings and behavior.

Task oriented therapy

This will help individuals to gain tool that will help them to change their behavior (Often feelings).

Experience oriented

These attempts will increase on experience that will help growth and personal development.

Group Psychotherapy

It is a treatment modality in which selected group of clients are treated by a qualified group therapist. The goal of group therapy is to alleviate their psychic system, to reduce anxiety and to providing clients with opportunities to modify and list new behavior in a controlled setting.

Two types of groups are discussed here.

Therapy Groups

Groups of persons come together to receive psychotherapy in a group settling.

Supportive Groups

Group of persons that come together for the primary purpose of offering support education and/or socialization/recreation.

The members of the group are usually strangers coming together for some purpose. There will be a group leader or facilitator or group therapist, the person who select group member according to purpose and goals of the group, the group may be homogeneous or heterogeneous.

A group can also be an open group or closed group.

An open group is one where participants may come and go depending on their individual needs.

These groups are common on inpatient wards and self help groups.

A closed group begins with a certain number of participants and is not open to new members. They are often found in outpatient settings often have a focus on psychotherapy.

Advantages of Group Therapy: (Valoms Goals of Groups Therapy 1985)

Instillation of Hope

Progress of others in the group is observed by a group member and he will be hopeful about receiving similar help.

Universality

A group member observes that others also share similar feelings, have similar problems. Therefore, anxiety is reduced.

Imparting of Information

During group meeting, many informations relating, medications and other problem solving techniques are shared among personal.

Altruism

The opportunity to support and help others will give increased self-esteem. It is also encourages a preoccupied individual to become less self focused.

Imitative Behavior

The group leader or a group member who has already mastered a particular psychosocial skill can be a valuable role model.

Interpersonal Learning

The group offers varied opportunities in relating to other people. Group members list new ways of relating in a safe environment.

Catharsis

An out pouring of emotional tension through verbalization or display of feelings may occur in a group session. This may be a tension reducing and growth enhancing phenomenon.

Preparation of Group Leader/Facilitator

The educational and experimental background for group leader depends upon the purpose of the group. If the group is a therapy group, using a distinct psychological, theoretical model, the nurse should be at graduate level and has experience in group therapy. It is important to note that the American Nurses Association (ANA) statement on scope and standards of practice for psychiatric/Mental health clinical nursing practice requires that nurses functioning as group therapist be master's prepared clinical nurse specialist (2000).

Nurse need not to be an advanced practice role to provide care to client to supportive group like.

Socialization group, recreational group educational group, reality orientation group, reminiscence group, and self help group, etc.

The group leader performs several tasks that facilitates group program. They are:
- Provides feedback and suggestion
- Elicit responses from silent members
- Clarifies verbalized thoughts and ideas as well as nonverbal communications
- Facilitates expression of feelings and concerns
- Reflects the feelings of the group
- Observes group behaviors
- Summarise progress and accomplishments
- Prepares the group for feelings associated with ending membership in the group
- Facilitates planning of future goals.

NURSES RESPONSIBILITY

1. Selecting members according to the purpose of the group.
2. Arranging time, frequency and place for group meetings.
3. Establishing group rules.
4. Negotiating contracts with group members.
5. Provide and maintain confidentiality among group members.
6. Intervene the group by means of communication skill role modeling, managing monopolizes.

Management of members anxieties, and facilitate the group towards establishment of goal.

Keep record of written notes of group sessions which included description of group its purpose, attendance, goals and composition. Pattern of group interaction, leadership, technique used, etc.

Family Therapy

The focus of intervention is not on the individual but on the family as a unit. Several family members take part in the therapy program. Both parents with the children whose problem brought the family for treatment. The aim of the treatment is to alternate the problems that led to the disorder. There are several varieties of family therapies in the patients.

Based on psychodynamic or behavior principles, the components of therapy may include problem solving, training in communicating techniques, writing a behavioral contact, and homework assign. Skynna (1069) suggest that conjoint family therapy is most useful when the parents cannot cope with the behavior of a child or adolescent or when a family makes one member a targetted for its problem.

Marital Therapy

Marital therapy given to both partners in a marriage. This is also called 'Couple therapy' sometimes used to include people living in common law of cohabitation.

This therapy is chosen when marital conflicts appears to be the cause of emotional disorder in one of the partner. There are various methods used like analytic method, transactional method, behavioral method and eclectic method, etc.

There are strong evidence that marital therapy is better than many treatment modalities and that the behavioral forms of martial therapy improves 60 percent of cases.

Social Therapy

The mentally-ill patients are often unable to participate acceptably in the prevailing social order. His illness is usually the result of an accumulation of social maladjustments rather than a single great catastrophe.

He lives a large extent into world of her own making, which may not be in reality. Therefore, it is the hospital responsibility to provide treatment which will help him to accept his social obligation and become a contributing member of society. To provide this treatment the hospitals should include various programs and social activities which will help the patient to accept his environment, adjust his environment and contribute to his own and other persons well-being.

The social therapy is defined as "organized group living in which integration and continuity of work, play and social activities produce a meaningful total life experiences in which the growth of individual capacity, to enjoy life, has maximum opportunity". The social therapy is to raise the quality of the individual lives, to provide more challenges and stimuli and to re-establish connections with the family outside. In general, the social therapy can introduce the principles of activity, freedom and responsibility and then help to work towards rehabilitation and the independent life.

Types of Social Therapy

1. Milieu therapy
2. Activity therapy which includes various therapies like occupational therapy, recreational therapy, music therapy, dance therapy, etc.

Milieu Therapy

It is Aimed at manipulating the environment in such a way that the individual can have positive emotional experience. Here the client is immersed in a carefully designed residential community in the purpose of learning new patterns of interpersonal relationship.

Three important components in milieu therapy are:
1. Physical setting.
2. Rules and ritual of the setting
3. Staff members > attitude and behavior
   The client best suited in milieu therapy are:
1. People whose behavior is violent and distractive and needs external control
2. People with deficits in ego function, such as reality closeup testing and problem solving. Who are so disintegrated that they need continuous support and care.
3. People in crisis, need change from their customary environment into a structured and protective one.

This therapy has evolved from the therapeutic community approach planned by Maxwell Jones.

2. Activity Therapy/Work/Occupational Therapy

Occupational therapy is the treatment of man in the totality, through his active participation in purposeful activity. The use of purposeful activity helps, provide a realistic environment to the patient and guides his perception of himself and the environment.

Occupational therapy also described as an active method of treatment with profound psychological justification (Clark 1963).

The origin and introduction of occupational therapy was to the period following the so called 'dark ages' in the year 1250 AD Hospitals were setup through without much attention to the mentally-ill. Attention was directed to analysis of movement. Occupational exercises and activities for toughening-up and recreations were recommended by physicians.

In 1752, activity therapy was established in USA, where the use of occupation as treatment for the mentally-ill continued to develop. Until the civil war in 1860.

In 20th century Adolf Mayer a Neuropathologist developed occupational therapy and reported that proper use of time in some helpful activity appeared as fundamental issue in the treatment of Neuropsychiatric patient. In 1905, Susan E Tracy, a nurse and the first practicing occupational therapist, noted the benefit of OT in relieving nervous tension.

DEFINITION

Occupation is defined as an activity which engages a persons resources of time, and energy and is composed of skills and values (Reed & Sanderson 1980).

Occupational therapy is defined as the art and science of directing a persons participations in selected activity to diminish or correct pathological problems and promote and maintain health (Engel hardt HT 1922).

Occupational therapy is used in different way.

As a means of assessment Assessment of his mental and physical competence and residual capacity. *Prospects* as whether the patient can return to his previous job or has to consider a new vocation can be deliberated with the help of OT

As a means of restoring general health and function So that patient's workhabit, general resistance to fatigue and efficiency is maintained enabling him to return to his work successfully.

As a means of restoring local functions In physical rehabilitation it involves joint mobility, muscle power, coordination and work endurance.

As a means of helping the permanently disabled To become independently developing areas of activities of daily living (ADL).

As a prophylactic measure Mainly by placing emphasis on exercise in maintaining general physical health and alleviation of depressions, anxiety and boredom.

Activities can be divided into the following categories:
- Creative activities, e.g. pottery, puppetry
- Commercial, e.g. typing, book-keeping
- Domestic, e.g. cooking home management
- Industrial, e.g. printing, assembly work
- Intellectual, e.g. solving crosswords/puzzles
- Recreation, e.g. games, dancing
- Those enriching social relationships of helping out the poor children, organizing functions for geriatric patients.

Advantages of Occupation Therapy

- It diverts the mind from morbid state
- It decreases his hallucinations as he concentrate on the activities
- It increases his socialization as he has to work with others
- It provides an incentive and goal
- Helps to maintain normal work habit
- Channelizes the psychomotor activities
- It enables to have a feeling of achievement
- It stimulates interest and attention
- Teaches social skills
- It increases self-esteem
- It helps the Rehabilitation with return of self-confidence
- It satisfies the emotional needs like, love acceptance and security through activities.

The therapeutic tools used in occupational therapy are the self, group and group activities, therapeutic milieu, creative and manual arts, recreational activities, library and educational activities, leisure activities and domestic activities.

Occupation therapy differs for the short-stay and the long-stay patients. It differs from patient to patient. It is a treatment which is given under expert medical personal for mental psychological problems. The therapist should have a knowledge of the disease, disabilities of the patient before providing specific occupation for the patient.

Here are few activities suggested for patients

Neurotics In neurotics the emotional conflict is main problem rather than lack of work practice. Activities encouraging social responsibility which divert from pre-occupying thoughts are used. Finger painting and other activities cannot be used for OCD, patient whom the activity strengthen the need to wash hands.

Manic patients Manic patients to be given repetitive rhythmic activities without many decisions, where he can utilize his excessive energy in a productive and useful way.
- Too many process allow distraction
- Isolated activities are preferred as he may interferes with the work of others
- In the hospital, sweeping, swabbing, washing plates, weaving, washing clothes be given.

Depressive patients Activities should be short-term creative and interesting and in small encouraging groups. Activities in open air and physical exercise are very good.
For example, Horticulture, out door games.

Schizophrenics Emphasis should be on social skill training especially personal hygiene. Regular exercise and work involving simple graded task with less decision making to be given. Small group activities are indicated which facilitate communication and interpersonal relationship.

Addicts Constructive work, which fosters and raises patient image and confidence in the minds of others are used. Industrial activities fostering specific talents are very useful.

MR Training in vocational and social skill to be given.

Occupational therapy is divided into two broad categories:
1. Activity therapy.
2. Vocational training.

Activity therapy Actual disturbing symptoms or needs are taken into consideration. It is not usually connected with the person's occupation.

For example, finger painting or clay work for regressed patients.

In vocational training The main aspect to be looked into are:
- Patients illness and its duration
- Past working experience
- Present interest of the patient
- Current mental status
- Family resources
- Current abilities of the patient.

Training Tips in Occupation Therapy for Patients

- Develop good interpersonal relationship
- Select a type of work depending upon his experience, interest, mental and physical condition. Keeping in mind the families interest and resources

- Start with simple work in a comfortable environment
- Once one teaching has occurred give time for over learning
- Support and use various types of reinforces to motivate the patient
- Assess work behavior using work behavior assessment scale and reward him accordingly
- Educate patient and family members regarding. need and positive effect of work for the patient.

The value of work as a vehicle of social stimulation was clearly demonstrated in an experiment by wing and Freud Enberg (1961).

There was significant reduction in the patients social withdrawal and socially embarrassing behavior with work (EK danli 1966).

Art Therapy

Through history, art has been important means of expression. It was also recognized as a bridge between the clients inside and outside world.

Wilman saw art therapy as 'a way' to bring order out of chaos or choitic feelings and impulses with in Art therapy is defined as the use of creative art process to psychotherapy and rehabilitation.

The primary goals of art therapy are:

1. Provide a safe environment for the patient free of judgment and censorship in the expression of feelings and unconscious experiences.
2. Select a medium that will promote the therapeutic balance between regression and use of healthy defenses.
3. Encourage the client to verbally share there are art work with the therapist individually or with a group

to increase insight and promote interaction with others.

4. Provide a creative experience as an out let for emotion and perception.
5. Expose clients to art materials so that they may benefit from the creative effects of color and design.

The nurses role includes observing clients use of the art media, encouraging their verbal expressions about the artwork. Noting specific content of the artwork and its relationship to his life.

Recreation Therapy

Recreation can be thought of as creating again or refreshing oneself by some form of play, amusement or relaxation. Play is a powerful tool as it helps in ventilation, act out aggression, achieve motor mastery in children and recalling childhood success as adults.

Recreation therapy is defined by the American Therapeutic Recreational Association (1991) as, treatment services which restore immediate or rehabilitate in order to improve functioning and independence as well as reduce or eliminate the effect of illness or disability.

Nurses should organize recreational activities in the wards such as audiovisual programmes, cooking sessions, special outings to temples, garden, sight seeing, or ball games, etc. Nurse has to select the activity based on the treatment goal, patient ability, lifestyle tolerance in social involvement and interaction, etc.

The four primary goals of recreational therapy are:

1. Provide clients with structured normal activities of daily living.
2. Assist clients in developing leisure skills and interest suitable to their lifestyles.

3. Agument verbal psychotherapy and other activity therapies.
4. Observe client reactions and evidence of progression or regression.
5. The nurses role include providing promoting activities and interaction that foster independence, responsibility and problem solving skills.

Dance Therapy

Dance has been used throughout history;for celebration 'worship' mourning and healing. American Dance Therapy Association defines dance therapy as 'the psychotherapeutic use of movement as a process which furthers the emotional', cognitive and physical integration of the individual.

Nurse observe clients movements as they reflect psychologic difficulties then the therapist presents theme to alter movement thereby affecting emotions and cognition change. The flow of the sessions if established as nurse facilitates a clients spontaneous movements and connects them to the movements of other with other method as mirroring the actions, changing it or moving in opposite directions.

So nurses role here includes participation in the activity, observing encouraging with honest observation and promoting discussion when possible.

Music Therapy

Since eighteenth century music has been documented as effective healing. Music therapy is defined as the use of music in accomplishment of therapeutic aims. The restoration, maintenance, and improvement of mental and physical health.

The music may be recorded music, song writing movement and music instrument. The goal of the therapy is to:

1. It increase communication skills.
2. It helps in expression of feelings of patient who does not speak with others. Through music he expresses his aggressive feelings by singing loudly in the group song.
3. Improves self-esteem.
4. Reduces maladaptive (stereotypic, compulsive, self-abusive, disruptive behavior, etc.)
5. Increases interaction with others.
6. Increase attending behavior.
7. Improve fine and gross motor skills.
8. Improves auditory perception.

   The nurses role includes:
   - Organizing music program for the patient by the patients
   - Encourage patient to participate in music activities
   - Observe their nonverbal expression during music
   - Provide positive reward to participating in the program.

Psychodrama

Is the use of guided dramatic action to examine problems raised by an individual to clarify issues increase physical and emotional well-being enhance learning and develop new skills.

Phychodrama uses the dramatic technique to 'act out' the emotional problems. It allows increased awareness of the problems and an opportunity to actively work through them. Nurses role in psychodrama includes observing client's reactions and encouraging client to relate these reactivities to their own issues.

Complementary Modalities

There are several complementary modalities used in psychiatry mental health care. Each of the modalities and techniques described requires further study and in many cases certification as a practitioner to incorporate in to his practice.

Complementary modalities are those modalities being used as an adjucent to medical care and psychiatric treatment that are thought to have effect on sleep disturbance, anxiety, and other emotion.

The complimentary modalities

Relaxation: It is defined as a psychophysiological state characterized by parasympathetic dominance involving multiple. Visceral and somatic symptoms including absence of physical mental, and emotional tension (Kolkmier 1988).

Here one's level of consciousness moves from beta activity, which occurs when one is mentally alert and actively thinking, to alpha activity, a state that falls between full consciousness and unconsciousness (Dimollto 1981). The benefits of this alpha state include an increase in creativity, memory, and the ability to concentrate ultimately an improvement in adaptive functioning.

The term relaxation response was first used by Herbert Benson when referring to the psycho physiological state where muscles are relaxed, tension is released blood pressure, heart rate, and respiratory rates are decreased the brain is in alpha state and the parasympathetic system is activated. When the para-sympathetic systems are activated the person feels calm. The Alpha brain state is a deepened state of relaxation.

TECHNIQUES OF RELAXATION

Deep Breathing Exercises

Deep breathing is a simple technique that is basic to most other relaxation skills. Tension is released when the lungs are allowed to breath in as much oxygen as possible (Kames communication, 1988).

Breathing exercises have found to be effective in reducing anxiety, depression, irritability, muscular tension and fatigue (Davis, Eshelman a MC May, 1982).

This exercise should be practiced in few minutes three or four times a day or whenever a feeling of tension occurs.

Technique

1. Sit or stand or lie in a comfortable position, ensuing that spine is straight.
2. Place one hand on your abdomen and the other on your chest.
3. Inhale slowly and deeply through the nose, the abdomen should be expanding and pushing upon your hand. The chest should be moving only slightly.
4. When you have breathed in as much as possible, hold your breath in few seconds before exhaling.
5. Begin exhaling slowly through the mouth pursing your lips as if you were going pursing to lips helps to control how fast you exhale and helps airways open as long as possible.
6. Feel the abdomen deflate as the lungs are emptied of air.
7. Begin the inhale-exhale cycle again focus on the sound and feeling of your breathing as you become more and more relaxed.
8. Continue for 5 to 10 minutes at a time.

Progressive Muscle Relaxation (PMR)

Progressive muscle relaxation is a technique of alternately tensing and relaxing muscle groups throughout the body to become aware of tensions and the contrast between muscle tension and relaxation.

This method was developed in 1929 by Chicago physician Edmond Jocobson. Excellent results have been observed with this method in the treatment of muscular tension, anxiety, insomnia, depression, fatigue, irritable bowel, muscle spasms high BP, mild phobias stuttering, etc. (Davis et al 1982).

Each muscle grasp intensed for 5 to 7 seconds and then relaxed for 20 to 30 seconds during which time the individual concentrates on the difference in sensation between the two conditions. Soft slow background music may facilitate relaxation.

Other Relaxation Methods

Other relaxation method include countdown, eye muscle tightening and relaxing.

Countdown is a technique in which the client is advised to countdown slowly from 100- to 0 and feel both refreshed and relaxed when he reaches 0.

Eye muscle tightening and relaxing is done by instructing the client to focus intently on an object, which results in a certain amount of eye muscle tightening fatigue. He is then instructed to relieve the fatigue by closing the eye.

Guided Imagery

It is a technique builds on the relaxation and visual or other sensory images to enhance the relaxation and to prevent an image in the client that is one of healing.

Guided imaging is defined as an unconditional process in which the practioner leads the subject with specific words, suggestions, symbols, or images to elicit or positive resting (shames 1996).

It is also called pleasant memory technique. Here the patient is made comfortable and relaxed. He is told to close his eyes and is given suggestion to think back to an enjoyable event.

Lying on the sand, walking on seashore or man attractive past or asking the patient to think a special place where he has positive manner and experience being there and encourage the patient to express thoughts and feeling about the experience. Thinking of a pleasant event can bring many positive sensation to the patient.

This technique is used in:

- Clients undergoing medical procedures that one uncontrollable
- Maternity care, preparing for labor and childbirth
- Reducing depression
- Chemotherapy and cancer treatments
- To overcome drug addiction.

This technique cannot be recommended for panic disorder (cannot concentrate) psychotics or schizophrenias.

Hypnotherapy

Is a technique that involves varying degrees of suggestibility and a deep relaxation effect.

A trance like state is induced by the therapist or self-induced by the client. It is useful strategy for producing feelings of calmness, and tranquility and used as an antidote for anxiety disorder.

Hypnotherapy—the use of hypnosis to achieve resolution of psychic trauma and distress is used along with other forms of psychotherapy.

Hypnotherapy is also used in many areas of medical, dental and nursing practices. It is used:
- To gain relief from pain of various reasons
- During labor and delivery
- Managing migraine.

Massage and Touch

Massage is the stimulation of the skin and underlying tissues in the purpose of increasing circulation and inducing a relaxation response.

Therapeutic Touch (TT)

Therapeutic Touch (TT) is a specific technique developed in the 1970's by Krieiger (1979) at New york University of consists of only four steps process of Centering.
1. Assessing the clients-centering field.
2. Smoothing or unraffling the field.
3. Modulating (Transferring energy).
4. Knowing when to stop.

Pet Assisted Therapy

Animal assisted therapy is the purposeful care of animals to provide affection, attention, diversion and relaxation (Me doskey Bule chek 2000).

Pets particularly dogs, puppies and cats have been shown to decrease feelings of loneliness. So, it is used for patients to provide:
- Diversion
- Socialization
- And adjustment.

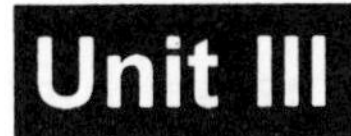

CHAPTER 10

Schizophrenia and Management

INTRODUCTION

Schizophrenia disorder are the commonest and if the social results consider, the most serious psychiatric disorder, many individuals start the symptoms in young age. This condition does not shorten the lifespan. As life advances this condition causes much chronic with negative symptoms and make the person more and more invalid and deteriorated in daily activities, i.e. will step to poor quality of life. If one look at the number of individuals coming to psychiatric out patient department, one can see a very good number is schizophrenias. These patients by virtue of their poor quality of life and progressive negative symptoms make the family members and society more and more anxious and unable to make themselves adjusted to care these individuals. Many eminent psychiatrist tried to understand schizophrenia. Many individuals who were studied for the cause were young and their symptoms had progressive deterioration. So, the eminent psychiatrist KREPLIN considered that this is one type of dementia, so he called this condition as dementia praecox. Later studies could served that those dimentic symptoms are not due to intellectual impairment, but it was observed that the loss of integration of various mental functions especially of affect and thinking. In schizophrenic the ideas held may be accompanied by an inadequate and inappropriate expression of feelings. This is why a Swiss psychiatrist E Bleuler coined the term schizophrenia means "splitting of mind". (Schizo—mind, phrenia—splitting)? (Handbook of psychiatric nursing by BRAIN ACKNER, 4th Edition, London, 1964).

DEFINITION

Of all psychiatric syndromes schizophrenia is the most difficult condition to define or describe. The main reason for the difficulty is that over a century many divergent concepts of schizophrenia have been described in different countries by different psychiatrists. Main difference of opinion persist till recent years. So, better to start with a simple comparison between two concepts in acute schizophrenia and chronic schizophrenia.

One of the simple *definition* is "It is a group of mental illness characterized by specific psychological symptoms leading to a disorganization of the personality of an individual. The symptoms chiefly interfere with the patients, thinking, emotion and behavior."

In acute schizophrenia the predominant features are delusions, hallucinations and interferences with thinking. Then features are otherwise called positive symptoms. Some individuals recover from these symptoms completely. But others progress to chronic symptoms. The chronic symptoms are usually apathy, lack of drive, slowness. These features are called negative symptom from which the complete recovery is questionable.

Epidemiology/Incidence

Schizophrenia is equally prevalent in men and women and its incidence is estimated in between 0.5 to 1.5

percent in adults. According to the World Mental Health Report 2001, 24 million people world wild suffer from Schizophrenia. It is prevalent across all socio cultural and national boundaries with a few exceptions in the prevalence rate in some and isolated communities. But the report of incidences can vary because of the differences in the diagnosis criteria in different countries. To conclude the incidences are always alarming when its effects in the society is considered.

Etiology

The exact cause is still not known. But there are theories to support the following factors as causes for schizophrenia:

Hereditary/genetic These are studies done on uni-ovular and bioovular twins to establish the hereditary factor of this disease.

Environmental factors The studies on adapted children of schizophrenia parents and vice versa have suggested the side of environment in these individuals with schizophrenia.

Endocrine factors Endocrine glands have direct or indirect control on the production and utilization of neurochemical substances. The imbalance of these neurochemical substances is behind to the causes of some behavioral problems.

Neurological/Neurochemical factors Thickening of corpus collosum, atrophy of cerebellum, enlargement of ventricle in brain are seen in schizophrenia patients.

Neuropathology Patient with chronic temporal lobe epilepsy have an increased risk of developing, schizophrenic symptoms and also in individuals with Huntington's chorea. There are incidences of schizophrenia after a brain injury. Electrical activity of the brain and the cerebral blood flow also can be related to symptoms of schizophrenia.

Psychodynamic Factors

According to Fraud in the first stage of libido was withdrawn from external objects and attached to the ego. The result was exaggerated self-importance of libidos made the external world meaningless, the patient attempted to restore meaning by developing abnormal beliefs. Malanie KLIEN believed that the origins of schizophrenia were in infancy. He told that the child could not identify the good or bad which may become the basis of later development of schizophrenia.

Family Factors

The psychological abnormalities in mother can cause for the schizophrenia behavior in children (Alahen 1958, 1970). Marital state in which one parent yielded to others eccentricities which dominated the family and marital schism in which the parents maintained contrary views so that the child had divided loyalties were also reported have contributions towards schizophrenic individuals.

Disordered communication in the family can be the cause for schizophrenia symptoms. Batson et al (1950) called it as double bind which is said to occur when an instruction is given overtly but contraindicted by a second more covert instruction. For example, a mother calls her child to come to her, but conveying by manner and the tone of voice that she rejects him. These double bind communication seems to be later makes the child unable to have correct thinking and effect.

Social Factors

The countries with contrasting culture can influence the thinking of people. The countries with cultures that do not differ much has lower incidence rate of schizophrenia. But where differences in culture are more the incidences of schizophrenia is reported higher. (Hollings head + Redlich 1958).

Some studies suggest that prevalence of schizophrenia to be highest in the low socioeconomic groups.

Migration, social isolation also are reported to be the causes of schizophrenia.

Precipitating Factors

Physical illness and childbearing, psychosocial stress, loss of job, loss of dear ones, unexpected financial loss) also can be precipitating factors of schizophrenia.

Subtypes of schizophrenia

1. Simple schizophrenia.
2. Hebephrenie schizophrenia.
3. Paranoid schizophrenia.
4. Catatonic schizophrenia.
5. Residual schizophrenia.
6. Un-differentiated schizophrenia.
7. Schizophrenia like disorder.

Simple Schizophrenia

Though it is called simple it is difficult to diagnose. It is characterized by early onset (in younger age), very insidious and may be arrested its own or may be progressive. The symptom may be marked social withdrawal. Shallow emotional response with loss of initiative and drive, wandering aimlessly, etc. Hallucination and delusion or usually absent, if present they are short-living and poorly systemized. As a whole prognosis is very poor.

Hebephrenia/Schizophrenia

Young people are more affected symptoms are more obvious. Hallucination and delusions are present. Smiling giggling to self is common. Mannerisms, gazing, blunting are seen, poor personal hygiene, impaired social and occupational functions are reported.

Prognosis is poor, but it may depend upon the pre-morbid personality and the ability to adjust to the adverse situations.

Paranoid Schizophrenia

Along with general symptoms of schizophrenia, paranoid schizophrenia has some special features. They are delusions of persecution, reference, grandiose, control, infidelity or jealousy. The delusions will be well systemized and well-connected with each other. The hallucinations also usually have persecutory in nature.

Disturbances of affect and speech also seen. The prognosis is better if treated in time and with correct doses of drug.

Catatonic Schizophrenia

It is characterized by marked disturbances in motor behavior. It can be in two forms.

Excited catatonia It shows increased motor activity ranging from restlessness, agitation, excitement, and aggression, etc. Increase in speech with increase pressure of speech, tonic of speech loosening of association and incoherence also are present.

All these behaviors are a result of delusions and hallucinations. Due to increase activities the individual may not eat or during which can have bad to severe dehydration, and malnutrition; if not treated the condition can lead to death.

Stupors (retarded) catatonia This is marked by extreme retardation of psychomotor activity. Mutism, rigidity, posturing, echolalia, echopraxia, negativism, waxy flexibility are the common symptoms. Mannerism, stereotypics also manifested casualy. Because of these symptoms the individual cannot eat or drink and can go to dehydration, malnutrition and death. Lack of motor activity soiling the cloth with motion and urine also seen. All the features may not be present at a time.

Residual Schizophrenia

As the term denotes when these active symptoms are reduced but not completely free, then it is called residual schizophrenia.

Undifferential Schizophrenia

When the symptoms are not meeting the symptoms of any above said type of schizophrenia, it is called un-differential schizophrenia.

Schizophrenic Like Disorder

Whatever definition of schizophrenia is adopted there will be a cause. There will be cases that resemble schizophrenia in some respects and yet do not meet all criteria for diagnosis. These disorders are grouped in to four groups.

    a.   Delusional or paranoid disorders.
    b.   Brief disorders.
    c.   Disorders accompanied by prominent affective symptoms.

d. Disorders without all the required symptoms for schizophrenia.

Clinical Manifestation

Symptom of schizophrenia are many and varying from time to time. They also depend upon the subtypes of schizophrenia. During acute stage to the symptoms are more active or positive in nature but when it turns to chronic the symptoms also turn to more passive or negative in nature. For convenient grouping the symptoms can be grouped as follows:

Disturbance of thinking

Stream
- Incoherence
- Flight of ideas
- Thought block.

Content-irrelevant
- Circumstantiality
- Neologism
- Delusions of persecution
- Echolalia
- Loosening of association
- Word salad
- Echopraxia.

Disturbances in Emotion
- Blunting/flattened affect
- Apathy
- Incongruence.

Disturbances in Behavior
- Violence
- Abusive
- Assaultive

- Diskinetive
- Agitative
- Bizarre.

Disturbances in Perception

- *Hallucination—Auditory*
  - Olfactory
  - Gustatory
  - Visual
  - Tactile
  - illusions

Disturbance of Attention

- Excessive day-dreaming
- Fantacy
- Spells of laughter
- Crying without reasons

Social Symptoms

Poor pen relationships
- Low interest in hobbies
- Poor appearance
- Attention deficits.

Other symptoms—Mannerisms

- Grimacing, gestures
- Catatonic features

Diagnosis

Diagnosis is done by taking history and repeated mental status examination.

Management

Management can be discussed under following headings:

Hospitalisation

Hospitalisation is necessary in different stages of acute symptoms with positive or negative symptoms. The indications of hospitalisation may be:

- Suicidal ideas
- Homicidal tendency
- Significant confusion
- Severe catatonic symptoms.

Drugs

a. Antipsychotics to reduce the imbalance of neuro-chemical imbalance.
   For example, Chlorpremazene, Clozapine, Resperidine, Olanzapine, Haloperidol, etc.
b. Benzodiazepines to reduce the anxiety and agitation.
c. Lithium to reduce the sehizo affective symptoms.
d. Antidepressant of those are symptoms of depression secondary to schizophrenia.

Electroconvulsive Therapy It is been indicated in

- Acute psychosis
- Catatonic symptoms
- Suicidal tendencies
- Not responding to drugs.

Group Therapy It is indicated when acute symptoms are subsided. This is useful to improve:

- Communication skills
- Problem solving skills
- Activities of daily living, etc.

Individual Therapy It is mainly supportive, and also analytic in nature to know the causes of denoted behavior and help the individual to avoid the situations. These are not effective unless the drug therapy is coined with.

Nursing Care of Patients with Schizophrenia

Patients with Schizophrenia will have the following problems:

Table 10.1: Nursing care of patients with schizophrenia

Sl.No	Problems	Objectives
1.	Withdrawn behavior	To promote socialization
2.	Nutritional problem	To promote adequate nutrition
3.	Insomnia	To promote adequate sleep
4.	Talking to self	To decrease talking to self
5.	Phantasy	To create reality world
6.	Delusion	To decrease delusion
7.	Auditory hallucination	To decrease hallucination
8.	Lack of personal hygiene	To promote hygiene
9.	Low self-esteem	To increase self-esteem.
10.	Impaired communication	To improve communication
11.	Self care deficits	To provide physical care

In general, the nursing care consists of:

1. Providing Therapeutic Environment

These patients are withdrawn, indifference to the surroundings, apathetic, like to sit alone and day-dream, so the environment around him should help him to come out of his symptoms and able to lose his negative attitude towards himself and rebuilt a new perception in its place.

- Provide stimulating environment with music, and clean cheerful physical setup with various activity which stimulates the patient on pleasant level of reality.
- Provide safe secured feeling: To provide this the routine of the ward activities should be scheduled and it should go as per the schedule.
- All the staffs attitude towards the patients should be consistent and treat the patients as an individual with dignity.

- The routines should make reasonable expectation from the patients.
- Control the noise and excessive light which may enhance his perceptual drugs function.

2. Develop Good Interpersonal Relationship with the Patients

- These clients will have difficulty in establishing trust with anybody and it is believed that problem started with the infant mother relationship.
- So develop a trusting relationship with the client. It needs lot of hard work and patients from the nurse as the patients needs a long periods of testing out before he trust the nurse.
- First develop 1:1 relationship with the patients then slowly he can start relationship with other. Everyday spend some time with the patients even if he is unable to respond verbally or in a coherent manner. This conveys the caring and interest which helps in development of trusting relationship.
- Be sincere and truthful.
- Give promises which can be realistically fulfilled.
- Give attention and positive feedback for acceptable behavior.
- Avoid appearance of rejection while interacting with the patients.

3. Communication Use simple, short sentences and specific words while talking with these withdrawn patients.

- Pay attention to his nonverbal communications, i.e tone, rhythm, gestures, body movements, etc.
- Use nonverbal communication appropriately avoiding any cause for misinterpretation, e.g: Touch may be misinterpreted in paranoid patients.

4. Take Care of Physical Needs

Because of lack of interest in the environment and prolonged regression patients will be unable to take care of their physical needs.

Personal Hygiene

- Assess of the patient level of functioning
- Motivate and encourage the patient to take care of himself
- Supervise the patients bath, mouth care and assist if necessary
- Give supportive comments and sincere praise when he does it.

5. Nutrition and Elimination

- Assess fluid and food intake
- Provide meals and supervise while eating
- Provide food in a group setting if patients is having suspicious behavior
- Find out the like and dislikes of the person before this illness and serve the food keeping these in mind.

6. Sleep

- Observe the pattern sleep.
- Provide all the nursing measures (Chapter 28) to provide good sleep for the patients.

7. Prevention of self harming and harming to other.

- Patients may have impulsive behaviors and have sudden attack on others with or without any provocation.

This may be due to their delusions

- Sometimes these patients may have to be protected from patient who are very aggressive and excited
- They should be constant observation of their behavior. If there is any agitation or mounting of tension it should be taken care
- Encourage the patient to ventilate his feelings and take appropriate actions
- Do not allow the manic patients to take care of withdrawn patients as aggressive or manic patients do not have patients to deal with withdrawn behavior so the may assault them
- They also must be protected from their idleness and indulgence in phantacy
- Prevention of suicidal attempts may be another problem in some withdrawn patients
- Self limits on unaccepted behaviors
- Discourage competitive activities
- Protect when they are responding to their hallucinations.

8. Engage in Work

Patients should be encouraged to participate in some kind of work this will help in decreasing hallucinations and delusions also improves his self-esteem.

- Start with simple activity, which he can do easily (like paper bag making) and appreciate when he completes
- Find out his interest provide work in that area
- Activity in the open air will be very useful for these patients, e.g. Exercise in open air gardening, etc.

9. Improve his Self-esteem

- Low self-esteem is the main reason for not communicating and nonsocializing with other. So

improving patients self-esteem is responsibility of
the nurse working with schizophrenic
- Recognize the positive acts or strengths of the
  patients acknowledge it
- Nonverbally convey that he is worthy and lovable
  by
    - Listening to him
    - Giving importance whenever possible
- Respect his ideas
- Provide simple achievable work, when he finished
  appreciate him
    - For example, Helping other patients
    - Doing simple activity.

10. Improve Socialization

- Encourage the patients to participate in social
  group
- To begin with he may be placed with one-to-one
  similar patients then help him to need in small
  group and later larger group
- Should encourage to involve in recreational and
  spiritual activities which will help in diverting and
  supporting him.

11. Support During Convalescence

- When the patients are recovering and ready for
  discharge good reassurance to be given to return
  to the society. They should be encouraged to talk
  out their feelings about going home
- Find a place to live and a job if possible help him
  to make plans as to what he is going to do with
  himself.

12. Social Skill Training It is very important for the schizophrenic patients. These patients will be lacking in many of the social skills, necessary to live in the society.

- Training may be given in skill like:
  i. Communications
  ii. Cooking
  iii. Housekeeping/clearing
  iv. Budgeting
  v. Seeking job
  vi. Shopping, dressing and personal hygiene, etc.

13. Discharge Planning and Health Education

- Family should be prepared to accept him in the family
- Patients and family should be educated about the disease condition and need for long-term treatment
- Family should be educated and instructed to:
  - Follow the treatment in long-term
  - Take interest in patients, in what he is doing even it sound dull and repetition to you.
  - Assign small responsibilities.
  - It helps to booster his sense of worth let him feel that he is valuable and productive member of the family as any other
  - Encourage and support the patients
  - Supervise his activities
  - Appreciate even if it is a small task done by the patients
  - Avoid reactions and criticism
  - Watch for relapse, sleeplessness will be earliest sign of relapse for these patients

Encourage the family to join in "families of schizophrenic" group which is source of comfort and solace to one other.

Other nursing problems and its nursing management is discussed in a separate Chapter 28.

BIBLIOGRAPHY

1. Ms. K. Lalitha-'Mental health and psychiatric Nursing' Gajanana book publishers, 1995.
2. Oxford textbook of psychiatry 2nd edition, 1983.
3. Handbook for psychiatric nursing by BRAIN ACKNER - 9th edition London, 1964.
4. Mary Varghese Essentials of Psychiatric and Mental Health Nursing B.I.Churchill Living stone New Delhi, 1994.

CHAPTER 11

Mood Disorders or Affective Disorders

INTRODUCTION

The main reason for calling these disorders so because these disorders mainly affect the mood. In these disorders, the fundamental disturbances is a change in mood or effect usually to depression or to elation (mania). Affect is a short lived emotional response to an event whereas mood is a sustained and pervasive emotional response which colors the whole psychic life. So, depression and mania are mood disorders not affective disorders. Most of these disorder tend to be recurrent and the onset of individual episode is often related to stressful events or stimulation.

The terms mania and severe depression are usually used to denote the opposite ends of the affective spectrum and hypomania is used to denote and intermediate state without delusions, hallucinations or complete disruption of normal activities.

TYPES OF DISORDERS

The affective disorders are divided into the following types:
- Mania—Unipolar

- Depression—Unipolar
- Mania—Depression/Bipolar affective disorder.

1. Mania—Unipolar

When the symptoms of mania occur in one individual once in life forms or separately it is called mania-Unipolar. It can be represented as:

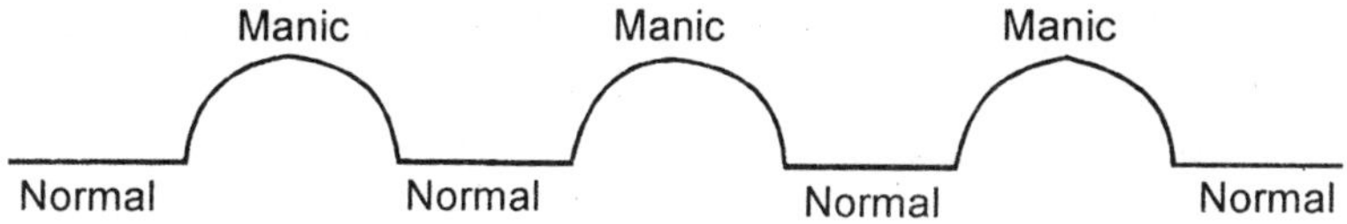

That means between each episode the individual becomes normal in his behavior.

2. Depression—Unipolar

When the symptoms of depression occurs in an individual once or recurs repeatedly it is called depression unipolar.

It can be represented as:

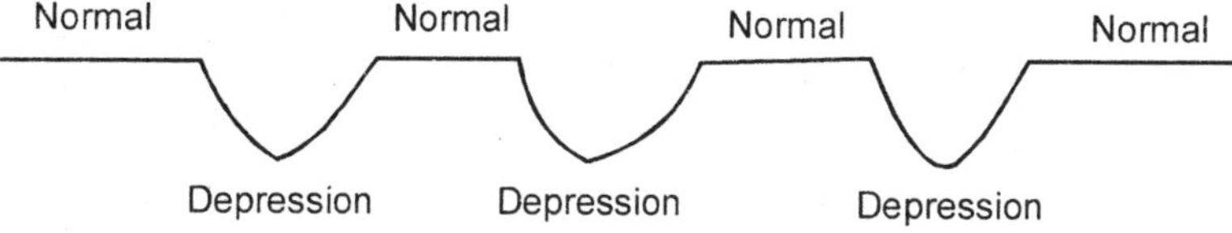

That means in between the episodes the individual behaves normally.

3. Bipolar affective disorders (BPAD)

It is cyclic in nature. In the individual has the symptoms of mania and depression intermittently. It can be represented as:

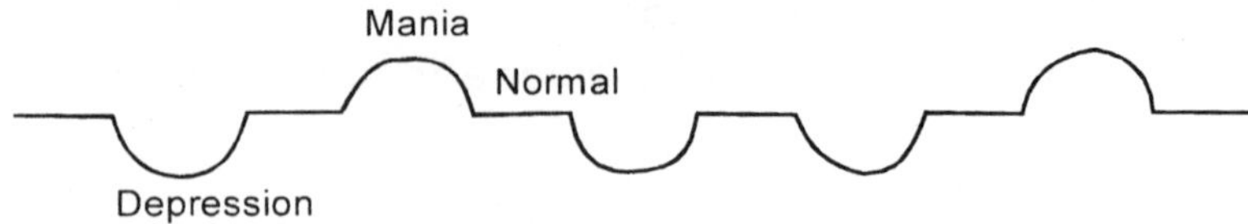

In between the both mania and depression episodes the individual may or may not touch the normality. Because of these manifestations it is difficult to give the etiology of both mania and depression separately.

Etiology of Affective Disorders

There are many different approaches to the etiology of affective disorder. Main consideration is the role of genetic factors followed by childhood experience stress factors, psychological and biochemical factors also are proved to be responsible for affective disorder partially.

Genetic Causes

Genetic causes are studied in moderate to severe cases of affective disorder. Most family studies have shown that parents, siblings and children of affective patients have a morbid risk of 10 to 15 percent as against 1 to 2 percent in general population. Twin studies and studies in adopted children also found on favor of the role of genetic factors as cause of affective disorders.

Psychological Causes

Loss of dear ones, learned helplessness and depressive cognition in childhood are suggested to be the cause of depressive disorders. The inferiority developed in young age also is suggested as cause of mania. But these are contradictory reports on several studies which intended to prove these causes.

Biochemical Causes

Again there are many hypothesis about the biochemical causes of affective disorders. It is suggested that three monoamine transmitters have been implicated. They are 5-hydroxytopamine (5.HT), noradrenaline and dopamine. The metabolism of these neurotransmitters are changed in the patient with affective disorder. But it is difficult to demonstrate that whether the life event affects these metabolisms then the individual starts symptoms or the changed metabolism affects the behavior.

Endocrine Causes

It is important to note the patients with endocrine disorder (Cushing's syndrome) develops depressive symptoms. It also is observed that depressive episodes are seen during menopause and after childbirth where there is a change in endocrine function. So, these are reasons to believe that endocrine glands have a role to keep the person normal in behavior and the change in the endocrine system can cause symptoms of depression or mania.

Water and Electrolytes Causes

The residual sodium has been reported high in both depression and mania. This plays an important role in nerve conduction which can be partially responsible for manic or depressive behavior. But it is the early to make a hypothesis on this regard.

MANIA

Mania is an affective disorder with consistent elevated mood with increased physical and mental activity present in an individual at least for few days or a week. When the mood is elevated that person seems to be cheerful optimistic, irritable easily become violent.

Manic types are classified into three stages.
1. Hypomania.
2. Acute Mania.
3. Delirious mania.

Hypomania

It is a mild form of mania. Patient will have moderate elation of mood and over activity. Energy is moderately increased. Thinking speeded up, delusions of grandiosity may be present. Patients will be mischievous, socially aggressive, argumentative, spends money extravagantly, appears bright, intelligent but intolerant to criticisms.

Acute Mania

The signs and symptoms are moderately increased.
- Mood shows excitement, he sings and dances, will have flight of ideas with rhyming, playing with words, etc. stream of thinking is increased.
- He may be demanding, revengeful and arrogant.
- Delusion of grandiosity and paranoid is present.
- He will be overactive, violent and have motor excitement difficult to control.
- Appetite increased but may not have time to eat because of his overactivity. So, they lose weight.
- Attention span decreased become iritable with environmental disturbances. Judgment is markedly impaired.

Delirious Mania

Patients are very much excited they may be hallucinating, delusional and extremely dangerous. They are constantly with purposeless activities. Speech is incoherent. Without treatment they may die of exhaustion.

Clinical Manifestations of Mania

1. *General Appearances*—Because of elated mood patients will have cheerful, overactive physically and mentally, dressed attractively, irritable, easily turns violent.
2. *Speech*—rapid, flight of ideas present.
3. Sleep—is disturbed, wake up early in the morning with lot of energy.
4. Appetite over activity is increased, eats hurriedly without conventional manners.
5. *Sex*—Sexual desires are increased and behavior may become uninhibited. Women neglect precautions against pregnancy.
6. Delusions—These are usually of grandiose may vary in content often.
7. Hallucinations—also occur usually in the form of voices speaking to patient about his special powers, occasionally of visions with religious content.
8. Poor judgment involves in high-risk activity. For example, business investment.
9. Insight—Very often insight is absent and the patient ventures to practice his extraordinary, impractical ideas.

With all above said symptoms these individuals may become tired in later days because of their inability to take physical and mental rest. It also will be the result of less time to eat and sleep. They may also become shabby when there is no time to do the personal hygiene and grooming.

Mixed Affective State

It is a state where the individual can have both mania and depressive symptoms at the same time. These patients may be overactive and over-laxative but having prefondly depressive thoughts. Sometimes these manic individuals become intensively depressed for a few hours and go back to their original state of manner.

Manic Stupor

In this condition although the facial expression suggests elation he may be mute and immediate. They are not harmful to themselves or to others but gives no answer to the questions, smiles without cause.

Diagnosis

Diagnosis is made by details history taking and the mental status examination and also all the clinical symptoms lead to make the individual inefficient to perform the social responsibilities of daily life for few days or a week it can be called a manic episode.

Management

When the symptoms are sufficient to disturb himself and others hospitalisation is advised. If the individual is harmful to himself and others and having a tendency to run away from the hospital, the individual is kept in a closed pavilion. This is a part of therapeutic environment.

Drugs In acute stage drugs are administered, by intravenous injections supported by oral route. Once the acute stage is over the oral drugs are continued for a quite long-time.

Drugs are:

1. Antipsychotics
   - Chlorpromazine (100 mg/d)
   - Haloperidol (2-3 mg/d)
   - Triflupromazine (5 mg/d)
2. Lithium is used in the prevention and treatment of manic episode.
3. These drugs bring the symptoms of acute mania under rapid control then doses are gradually increased.

Nursing care of patients with Mania

Table 11.1: Nursing care of patient with mania

Sl.No	Nursing Problems	Objectives
1.	Hyperactivity	To utilize the extra energy for constructive or productive work.
2.	Sleeplessness	To promote sleep.
3.	Nutritional problem	To promote adequate nutritrion.
4.	Lack of personal hygiene	To promote personal hygiene.
5.	Aggressiveness	To decrease aggression.
6.	Demanding	To reduce demanding.
7.	Grandeur delusions	To lessoss the delusion.
8.	Irritability	To reduce irritability.
9.	Flight of ideas	To decrease flight idea

GENERAL NURSING CARE

It consists of:

Maintaining Good Therapeutic Environment

- Since manic patients are hyperactive, talkative, irritable and angry, it is important to provide an unchallenging and nonstimulating environment. His ability to deal with stimuli may be impaired
- Stimuli of any forms, e.g.: excessive noise, bright colors, blearing TV or irritating personal should be avoided

- Separate rooms may be ideal with simple furnishing. Because of impulsive behaviors they may use the furniture destructively
- Provide a consistent and structured environment
- Respond to the clues of increased restlessness or agitation and remove the stimuli or isolate the patient
- Environment kept free from sharp and movable objects to avoid the self harm and harm to others.

Maintain Good Interpersonal Relationship (IPR)

- It is very easy to develop good IPR with these patients
- Use a firm, yet can relaxed approach, where his request being denied
- Use simple and short conversation. Avoid complicated ideas and long explanations and discussions
- Avoid comparison of his behavior with others
- Make only those promises which can be realistically fulfilled. Because breaking a promise will result in the development of mistrust which is detrimental to a therapeutic relationship
- Keep consistency with the patient most of the time
- Help the patients to identify his feelings and express it in an acceptable way and give positive feedback and reinforcement
- Set limits for his behavior if he has hyperverbal activity.

Promote Compliance with Drug Therapy

- Patients may be irregular in taking medicines, because of their hyperactivity and flight of idea. So, see that drugs are given in time
- Sedatives may be given if patient becomes aggressive or violent

- Check the report of the lithium level if the patient is on lithium carbonate. Reduce salt in diet if he is on lithium.

Promote Safety and Protection

- Recognize the mounting tension and anxiety as indicated by voice changes, muscle sins of tension, and increasing irritation. Take action to avoid possible injury to other and sedate him when you think he is going to be excited. Yet firm approach with the patients
- Maintain calm, supportive, yet firm approach with the patients
- Have constant observation on elated patients
- Avoid argument or challenges with excited patients
- Remove sharp instrument, broken glasses in the windows stick, rods or stones in the environment
- Do not allow elated patients to take care of depressed patient as these patients do not have patience and can harm depressed patients
- Sedate him whenever necessary.

Meeting the Physical Needs of Patients

- *Nutrition and elimination:* Here the patients are overactive needs lot of calories/they are too busy to eat, easily distracted during mealtime
- Monitor the patient's eating pattern, food and fluid intake because they may ignore feelings of thirst and hunger
- Provide high protein and high caloric diet with supplemental feedings
- Provide the patient with food that can be eaten on the 'run' (finger foods), e.g.: fruits, sandwich, etc. as they cannot sit, long-time to eat

- Provide frequent small feeds of easily digested food in order to slow down the metabolism
- Adequate fluid intake, regular toilet schedule, and adequate diet. Roughage should be given to avoid constipation
- When offering foods tell the patient that he has something to eat, instead of asking whether he like to eat or not
- Monitor patients elimination patterns.

Sleep

- Observe the sleeping pattern
- Use comfort and nursing measures to provide proper sleep
- Sedate if necessary.

Personal hygiene
- Patient is too busy to attend to the details of bathing brushing the teeth, shaving, etc. So supervise his personal hygiene
- Special attention to be given to the care of skin and oral hygiene.

Work

- Patients to be engaged in some kind of occupation. Especially for manic patients systematic continuous rhythmic activities where he can utilize his excessive energy in a useful or productive way to be given.
- Otherwise this excessive energy will be utilized in the destructive activities. For example, sweeping, swabbing, changing things, washing clothes, weaving, etc.
- Avoid highly competitive activity as it can exacerbates the patient's anger
- Observe for overexertion, if so, sedation may be necessary to control his behavior.

Involve the Patients in Recreational and Spiritual Activities

- Encourage the patients to participate in the common recreational and spiritual activities. For example, play, watching TV, going to temples
- Participating religious functions, yoga, meditation, etc.

Improve Self Esteem

Positive reinforcement to be given whenever possible.

Convalescence/Discharge Planning

- Observe for the mood swings in the opposite direction during convalescent period
- Encourage the patient to identify his goals and expectation after discharge and provide proper direction
- Health education to patients and family regarding care of patient after discharge is necessary.

DEPRESSION

Depression is an affective disorder, is otherwise called depressive syndrome. It is because of their clinical presentations which are varied so much that cannot be described fully, so these disorders are grouped by their severity.

Clinical Manifestations

General Appearance

Looks dull, looks down, shoulders bent, head inclined, movements reduced, dress and grooming neglected.

Psychomotor Activities

Psychomotor activities are reduced or retarded. *Speech*—No speech or less production, delay in answering, pause in conversation.

Mood

Low and miserable some may try to divide their mood which makes the doctor to make a diagnosis.

Mood may be anxious also. It may turn into irritable and agitated. Lack of enjoyment and reduced energy also noted.

Sleep is Disturbed

Early morning awakening is a typical clinical manifestation. They wake up two or three hours before the patient's usual time and does not fall asleep again. He lies awake and broods over the coming pessimistic days, or past failures. Very few of them sleep excessively but wake up unfreshed. This is an important feature to make diagnosis.

Thoughts—may be always pessimistic may go with feeling of worthlessness feeling of guilt.

Suicidal ideas and attempt—will be present.

Appetite—Appetite may be poor and weight loss is obvious

Difficulty—in concentration, intelligence and memory impaired.

Delusions and hallucinations—also present in many individuals.

Feelings—of hopelessness, helplessness and worthlessness.

Some of these symptoms may be present in many individuals for one day or few days without disturbing their daily activities. When these symptoms disturb their daily routine of personal life or official then it is diagnosed as depressive disorders.

Agitated depression: It is a disorder whose agitation is prominent in a depressive disorder. This is a state of restlessness, where the individual is unable to relax.

Retarded Depression

This is a term denotes a depressant's disorder in which psychomotor retardation is the prominent symptom.

Depressive Stupur

In this condition slowing of movement and paucity of speech become prominent in depressive disorder.

Diagnosis

Diagnosis is made by the thorough history taking and mental status examination.

Management

If the patient is not able to perform his daily activities either personal or official or both the admission is advised. If the patient expresses suicide is an indication to admit in intensive care units where close observation is possible. Depressive stupor or catatonic syndrome of depressant episode where artificial feed or intravenous infusion is required also becomes an indication for admission in intensive care unit.

Drug therapy is always needed which comprises of drugs like:

1. A usally antidepressants like – Imipramine 75 to 50 mg 300 mg, SSRI like fluoxitine, citulopeam, may be

used in same areas when tricyclic and tetracyclic anti depressant are are not responded then monoamine oxidaze inhibitors are given.

ECT is advised in severe depression along with drugs. Other treatments for mood disorder other than drugs include somatic treatment psychotherapy social therapy, etc.

NURSING CARE

Nursing Care of Patients with Depression

Usual nursing problems in this patients are:

Table 11.2: Nursing care of patient's with depression

Sl.No	Nursing Problems	Objectives
1.	Insomnia	To Promote sleep
2.	Suicide	To protect patient from self-destruction.
3.	Lack of Food intake	To promote adequate nutrion.
4.	Low self-esteem	To raise self-esteem
5.	Dependency	To insist self-confidence.
6.	Withdrawn	Socialization.
7.	Under active	To promote patient activities.
8.	Ideas of worthlessness	To create self-confidence
9.	Feeling of guilt and sin	To decrease guilt feeling.
10.	Lack of personal hygiene	To promote personal hygiene

These objectives are met by the following nursing actions.

Maintain a Good Therapeutic Environment

- Accept the patient as they are encourage **them in** every activities of them
- Provide a well structured and consistent environment which will reassure the patient
- The environment must be clean slightly stimulating, like pleasant colored wall, colourful curtain, wall paintings, etc. which will help in elevation of his mood

- Provide a secure and safe environment. Hazardous instruments and excessive furniture should be avoided
- Support his opinion consistently.

Develop Good Interpersonal Relationship

- Call the patient by name and accept him as a person
- Spend time with him, though he does't speak
- Provide sincere concern to the patient and be empathetic understanding
- Give attention and positive feedback for acceptable and positive behavior
- Avoid comparing his behavior with other.

Provide Safety and Protection

- Depressed patients safety is the nurses priority
- Observe the patients for the clues of destructive behavior and prevent from self-harming
- For severely depressed patient mental status examination may be done daily or twice a day. It will help the nurse to find out any precipitating factors for the episode. If so it can be avoided with timely action.

Prevent Suicide/Self-harming

- Most of the depressed patients will have suicidal tendency or self-destructive behavior
- So assess if there is any suicidal or self-harming tendencies
- Spend some time with him talk to him and assess the level of suicidal ideas. Suicide is crying for help". People about their will be eagerly waiting to talk about then problems and want to get help

from others. Research indicates that people have given clues for their suicidal attempts before they committed suicide.

- Maintain close supervision of the patient
- Keep the environment free from potentially danger objects such as sharp instruments razor, blades, scissors, broken glass pieces, ampule files, etc. Hanging open wires should be removed. Broken glasses of window to be immediately replaced
- Routine safty check has to be done
- Provide hospital gowns rather than saree or pyjamas
- Search him and his belongings
- Patients should not be left alone, especially when he goes to bathroom
- Observe frequently or continuously on one-to-one basis
- Keep the ward drugs safely
- Never allow the patient to lock the door from inside
- Make the patient to ventilate his feelings. Discuss about his suicidal thoughts and plans that will help to reduce his anxiety
- Establish 'No suicidal' contract
- Explore patient's strengths like good achieve-ments and assets of him which will reinforce the feeling of useful and needed convey the feeling of acceptance and belonging. Every shift nurse should be aware about the suicidal risk patients
- Promote decision making and coping skills to the patient.

Take Care of His Physical Needs

Nutrition and Elimination
- Monitor patient eating pattern and food intake as most of the patient may starve or take inadequate food/because of their depressive feelings
- Be with him when he is eating
- Provide food according to his likes and dislikes
- Provide more fluids and roughage to prevent from constipation
- Maintain intake and output chart in seer depressive patients and record weekly weight
- Offer foods that requires little effort to eat
- Give positive feedback when the patient is taking food properly
- Observe and record the pattern of bowel limitation.

Sleep
- Most of the depressed patients will have less/decreased sleep
- Reassure the patient that you are around to help him which indicate the feeling of concern
- Provide quiet environment and comfortable bed to sleep
- Avoid daytime sleep and provide physical activity in the evening
- Limit coffee or stimulant during everyday and night
- If there is an psychological problem, make the patient to ventilate his feeling
- Use medications if necessary.

Physical Hygiene
- Assess patient level of functioning
- Help him to maintain his personal cleanliness which will enhance his self-esteem.

Engage in Activities

- Provide some activity for the patient. In the beginning unschedule or nonpurposeful activities also can be planned with the interest of avoiding depressive thoughts. Later more purposeful and scheduled activities may be planned
- Open air activities will be very helpful in the depressed patients. For example, Exercise in the open air, etc.
- Provide a very simple and achievable job in the beginning when he completes appreciate him
- Schedule his daily activities plan according to his interest
- Allow him to participate in group activities, initially small groups then the number can be increased.

Provide Recreation

- Know the patients hobbies, interest, etc. and involve him in various recreational activities
- Provide specific timings for recreational activities in daily schedule.

Meet His Religious Needs

- Encourage daily prayer and common prayer meeting as they will help in providing mental piece and satisfaction
- Allow time for yoga, medication, etc. in daily schedule.

Improve Self-esteem

- Low self-esteem is the main reason for these patients feeling of hopelessness, helplessness and worthlessness. So, create an atmosphere which can improve his self-esteem.

- Call the patient by name and show acceptance as a person.
- Help the patient to identify his strength/positive points.
- Give attention and positive feedback achievement in life.

Convalescence

- During convalescence period many depressed patients will have suicidal ideas.

Discharge Planning and Health Education

- Family should be involved in discharge planning.
- Health education should be given regarding.
  - Illness, course, cause, and duration treatment, etc.
  - Importance of regular medication.
- Identification of early symptoms of relapse.
- Patient should be helped to find a placement occupation, financial assistance, etc.

Many times an individual may go for manic and depressive episodes alternately. So, the relatives should be given knowledge of both manic and depressive episodes. They should be able to identify the early signs and symptoms of both manic and depressive episodes and instruct to report as early as possible. They should be instructed the medication given for mania in case the individual starts having symptoms of depression and vice versa, for that reason make them understand the importance of drug level in the blood frequently.

CHAPTER 12

Neurotic Disorder

INTRODUCTION

Psychosis is a term used to denote the major psychiatric disorders where the individual does not have the touch with reality. Neurosis is a word used to denote a group of behavioral problems that have three features in common. First point is these are functional disorders that is they are not accompanied by any organic disorder of the brain. Second point is, however severe is the condition the affected individual does not lose the touch with external reality. Third is, they differ from personality disorders, because they have a discrete onset rather than having a continuous development from early adulthood.

Etiology of Neurosis

Genetic Cause

Studies show that different types of neurotic conditions run through families and close relatives. Twin studies also shows considerable evidence that genetic cause of neurosis.

Influence of Childhood

Upbringing, neurotic traits in childhood, and neurotic syndromes in childhood may become the cause for neurosis in adulthood. There are studies in favor of this hypothesis, but some studies contradict to this.

Psychoanalytic Theory

Fraud talk that the etiology of neurosis have three components. He proposes that anxiety is the central symptom of all neurosis. Second is that the anxiety arises when the ego fails to deal the demands of and to satisfy the superego. Third point is that the neurosis originate in childhood, from a failure to pass normally through one or other of the three stages of development that is oral, anal and genital.

Faulty Learning

Different people suggest that learning theories propose mechanism by which experiences in childhood and in later life rise to neurosis. Some theories support the fraud's theory. They talk that repression causes, avoidance learning, emotional conflict. Second theory tells that anxiety is a drive state other symptoms are the learned behaviors to reduce this anxiety. There are many other studies which have positive and negative acceptance of faulty learning as a causes of neurosis.

Environmental Causes

Under this heading the subheadings are:

Poor living condition: There are studies to prove that people from poor living condition when they move to better housing colonies the rate of neurosis; has decreased.

Noise: People who always experience loud noise, e.g. those who live near big airport tend to develop neurosis condition later.

Working condition: The work which requires continuous attention but poor initiation or responsibility can cause neurosis.

Prolonged–unemployment: This also makes the man anxious and may go onto avoidance, somatic symptoms, etc.

Life Events

It is known that patients with one kind of neurosis report more life events in three months before the onset of the disorder. This may not be true in everybody's life. This depends upon their ability to adjust to the events, the meaning of these events in their life.

All the above said causes give a unpleased answer. It is that the biosociophysiological cause is the correct term to be the etiology of neurotic disorder.

DIFFERENT CONDITION IN NEUROSIS

Anxiety Disorders

Anxiety disorders are abnormal behavior which manifest physical and mental symptoms of anxiety and they do not come secondary to organic brain disease or to any other psychiatric disorder.

Clinical Manifestations

General appearance Look anxious, raised forehead, tense posture, skin may be pale, sweating of palm and feet especially, easily cries.

Psychological symptoms Less concentration, irritability, poor memory, sensitivity to noise.

Physical symptoms Dry mouth, difficulty in swallowing, epigastric discomfort, loose motions, palpitations, increased frequency of micturations, headache.

Phobic Anxiety Disorders

These phobic anxiety disorders have the same core symptoms as generalized anxiety disorders. Most of the time the individual is free from symptoms, but some special situations of phobia the individual experiences anxiety. These individual try to avoid situations which can provoke anxiety still, while avoiding these situations the individual experiences anxiety. These situation can be of a crowded place, objects, e.g. spider, cockroach, natural disasters like thunder. For clinical purposes all these phobias are divided into three categories:
  a. Simple phobia.
  b. Social phobia.
  c. Agoraphobia.

Simple Phobia

These are characterized by unappropriate fear of some situation or objects. Simple phobias are often characterized by adding the name of the stimulus, e.g. spider phobia, where the individual experiences anxiety to see a spider or he avoids the sight of spider.

Etiology of most phobias, in adult life is a continuation of childhood phobia. In childhood all phobias are normal. But in teenage they are overcome, leaving few as permanent in adult life. Psychoanalytic explanation is that phobias that persist are not related to the obvious stimulus but a hidden source of anxiety. Some of the phobias are continued because of a severe encounter with a particular situation. For example, fear of dogs because he had an extensive dog bite in the childhood.

Treatment

Behavioral therapy in different stage is the recommended treatment.

Social Phobia

This is a disorder where a person is inappropriately anxious in situations in which he is observed and could be criticized. Here the individual avoids these situation, if at all enters to these situations avoids conversation or try to isolate himself. It can start in early adult life without any cause. This may continue in different situations of same type. Social phobias are different from personality disorders, where the individual shows lifelong shyness and lack of self-confidence.

Etiology

Is not fully understood. It may be a combination of conditioning and abnormal cognition. In other words, it may be due to defective learning experience in childhood.

Treatment

Cognitive behavioral therapy is effective to correct the social phobia.

AGORAPHOBIA

In this phobia, the individual experiences when they are away from home, in large crowds. They also show the symptoms of depression, obsession thoughts, etc. Other symptoms like fear of bus, train, supermarkets, hairdresser, etc. This may start abruptly. It may be while waiting for bus, train, etc. An unknown fear, starts and continue everytime when the individual is put into the same situation.

Etiology

There are few theories to explain the etiology:
  i. It proposes unconscious mental conflicts related to unacceptable sexual or aggressive impulses.

ii. Learning mechanisms may be responsible to develop agoraphobia.

iii. Personality plays an important role in developing agoraphobia.

Treatment

Behavioral therapy is the recommended treatment.
Other phobias are:

i.   Phobia of dental treatment.
ii. Phobia of exertion.
iii. Phobia of vomiting.
iv. Phobia of flying.
v.   Phobia of space.

CONVERSION AND DISSOCIATE DISORDER/HYSTERIA

Until recently conversion and dissociate disorder were called as hysteria. Hysteria the term came from hystero —means uterus. The symptoms associated with hysteria were usually identified in women than men in early days. So, the eminent psychiatrist on these days corned the word hysteria for that group of symptoms.

Later the terminology is changed to conversion and dissociate disorder. It is mainly because of the word hysteria is used in everyday language to denote extravagant behavior and it is confusing to use the same word for the deferred aspect of this syndrome and also these symptoms are seen in men and women widely.

Etiology

Psychoanalytic Theory

Fraud and Blreuer (1895) explained hysteria suffer mainly from some reminescence that is from the effects of emotionally changed ideas logged in the unconscious at sometime in the past. Studies in the later years also explained the combined effects of repressions and the conversion of psychic energy into physical channels in some way in later years of life. These ideas are not explained or tested. Still this is widely accepted.

Genetic

These are studies to support the positive effect of heredity in the manifestation of conversion and dissociate disorders.

Stress as a Cause

There are studies to explain that these symptoms may be reaction of the nervous system to excessive stress. These reaction may subside quickly. But there are occasions this reaction can be prolonged in the ways. Firstly they may be deliberately cultivated by someone who wants to take advantage of the symptoms. Secondly, these mechanisms that frequently repeated become habitual. These theories also never been substantiated. But this gives the ideas of voluntary and involuntary causes of a conversion and dissociative symptoms.

Clinical Manifestations

Conversion and dissociate symptoms are not produced deliberately. But these individuals initiate the symptoms that he has seen directly. These disorders usually intend, to get some advantage which is called secondary gain.

Disorders of Movement

Paralyses
Disorders of gait
Tremors
Aphonia and mutism

Disorders of Sensation

Hyperesthesia
Psychogenic pain's
Blindness
Deafness
Convulsion
Nausea
Vomiting

Disorders of Intelligence/Memory

Amnesia
Stuper
Multiple personality

Diagnosis

Diagnosis is difficult because it may be close to the symptoms of some other conditions. The differential diagnoses are:
- Organic disease of nervous system like partial complex seizure
- Histrionic personality
- Malingering.

Management

Treatment is mainly behavioral therapies. They are abraction, psychotherapy. Other treatments modalations are meditation and yoga. These are supportive therapies, not permanent solution for these symptoms.

Other condition: They can be mentioned under neurosis are depersonalization and hypochondrias.

CHAPTER **13**

Anxiety Neurosis

INTRODUCTION

Anxiety is often thought of as an unpleasant feeling but it is a necessary evil. Anxiety motivates human being to tackle, situations and achieve goals of life. It can be explained as a form of tension or an uncomfortable feeling related to an impending doom and can be only observed from the behavior.

DEFINITION

Anxiety is universal primitive unpleasant feeling of tension and apprehension. It is a state where a person has strong feeling of worry or dread, when the source is nonspecific or unknown. It is experienced as a vague discomfort in its early stage, as the level of anxiety goes up, it may be experienced as disintegration of self, a diffuse apprehension, a profound by irrational experience or feeling of helplessness.

Anxiety is not the same as fear. Fear is a feeling around by a known and real danger and the intensity is according to the seriousness of danger.

DIFFERENCE BETWEEN ANXIETY AND FEAR

Anxiety: It is a state wherein a person feels a strong sense of dread, frequently accompanied by physical symptoms of increased heart rate, respiratory rate, elevated blood pleasure (Autonomic nervous system responses) without having a specific source or reason for his emotions.

Fear

It is a state wherein a person feels a strong sense of dread with autonomic nervous system responses that are focused on a specific object or event.

For example, fear of tornado

Fear of surgery

Fear of getting a job.

Both fear and anxiety are the same, only in the sense that both are reactions to threat and the physiological changes are similar as both reactions are triggered by release of adrenaline into blood in order to prepare the person to meet the real or imagined danger.

Causes of Anxiety

Anxiety results where there is threat to the security of the individual. Threat can be to the biological integrity or to the self system. Biological integrity, e.g., Impending interference with basic need such as food, water clothing, etc.

Self system: For example, Unmet expectation for oneself.

Unmet needs for status and prestige

Inability to gain self-respect, etc.

Symptoms of Anxiety

Genetic and neurochemical factors have been implicated in anxiety proneness. There are physical, affective, behavioral and cognitive symptoms in anxiety.

Physical Symptoms

These include
- Palpitations, hyperventilation, shortness of breath, dizziness, faintness, tremulousness, tightness in the throat
- Dilatation of the pupils, flushing of the skin, diaphoresis, excessive facial to palmer sweating
- Diarrhea, frequent urination, nausea muscular tension, sleep problems.

Affective Symptoms

- Tension uneasiness—increasing distress and pain, characterized by a sense of dread
- Sense of losing control
- Sense of impending insanity.

Behavioral Symptoms

- Restlessness that becomes agitation as the level of anxiety increases
- Inability to act on own behalf which increases as intensity of anxiety increases.

Cognitive Symptoms

Deterioration in perception, information processing, learning, problem solving and decision making.

Levels of Anxiety

Anxiety can be classified into mild, moderate, severe and extreme panic levels. In mild anxiety, the person experiences day-to-day tension and is alert with an increased peripheral field. In moderate anxiety, the person focuses only on the immediate concerns, with a narrowed peripheral field. In severe anxiety the persons, peripheral field is greatly reduced and to individual focuses on a specific detail. In a panic state the person has feelings of died or terror and is unable to control his behavior.

Mild Anxiety +

- Persons peripheral field is narrowed
  - Sees, hears, and grasps less but can attend to more if directed to do so
  - Decreased attention span
    Decreased ability to concentrate.

Moderate ++

- Persons peripheral field is narrowed
- Sees, hears, grasp less but can attend to more if directed to do so
- Decreased attention span
- Decreased ability to concentrate.

Severe +++

- Attention focused on the shattered details
- Pre-occupied with feeling of extreme discomfort
- Cognitive process such as reasoning:
  abstract thinking and problem solving are impaired.

Panic ++++

- Very poor concentration
- Perception is distorted
- Can not to focus on what is happening
- His perception of the environment is dangerous
- Behavior lacks cognitive control and becomes unpredictable.

Adaptation Responses on a Continuum of Anxiety

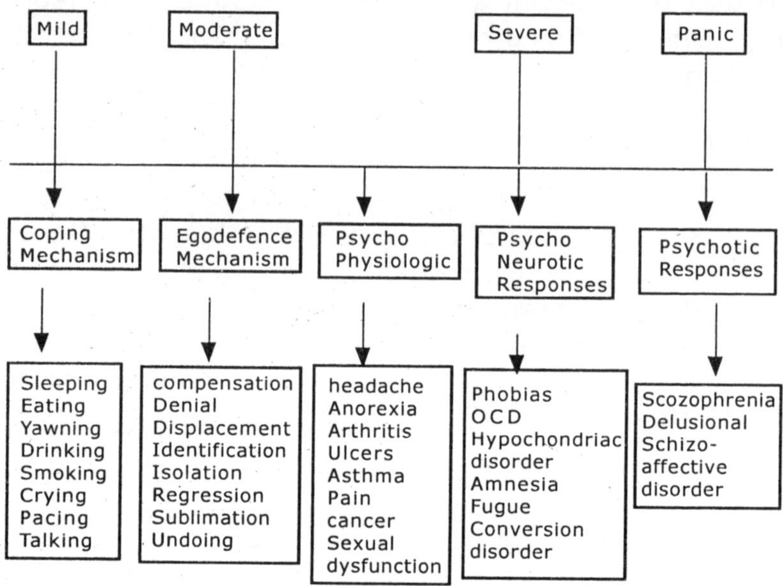

Mild Anxiety

Mild anxiety at the mild level individuals use a number of coping behavior that satisfy their needs and provide comfort. Menninger et al. (1963) described the following types of coping mechanism used by individuals to relieve their anxiety in stressful situations:

Sleeping	Drinking
Eating	Yawning
Crying	Day-dreaming
Smoking	Laughing
Pacing	Nail biting
Foot swinging	Talking to somebody to whom he feels comfortable

Physical exercise

An individual has his or her own unique ways to relieve anxiety.

1. Mild to Moderate Anxiety

As the level of anxiety increases, the ego strength is tested and energy is mobilized to control the threat. Anna Fraud (1953) identified a number of defense mechanisms used by the ego to face the threat to biological and psychological integrity. All these defense mechanisms are used either consciously or unconsciously as a protective device in ego in an effort to relieve mild to moderate tension. The defense mechanisms are unconscious processes whereby an individual handles unacceptable drives, thoughts, feelings, wishes by changing them into socially acceptable ones. These defense mechanisms will become maladaptive when they are used such an extreme degree that they distort reality, interfere with interpersonal relationships, one's ability to work productively and promote ego disintegration instead of self-integrity (Stuart and Sundeen 1987). The major defense mechanism identified by Anna fraud are:

- Compensation
- Denial
- Displacement
- Indentification
- Intellectualization
- Introjections, etc.

2. Moderate to Severe Disorders

Anxiety at moderate to severe level remains unresolved over an extended period of time can contribute to a number of physiological disorders. Common examples and psychophysiologic conditions are: migraine headache, angina pectoris, obesity, anorexia nervosa, bulimia, nervosa, rheumatoid arthritis, ulcerative colitis, gastric ulcers, asthma, muscle spasm, sexual dysfunction and cancer, etc.

3. Severe Anxiety

Extended periods and repressed severe anxiety can result in psychoneurotic disorders. They are:
1. Anxiety disorder.
2. Somato form disorder.
3. Dissociative disorder.

4. Panic Anxiety

At this extreme level of anxiety person is not capable of processing what is happening in the environment he may loose contact with reality. If it prolong for long-time psychosis occur which is defined as a gross disorganization of reality. Examples of psychotic responses to anxiety include the schizophrenia: schizo-affective and delusional disorder.

Types of Anxiety

There are four types of anxieties.
1. State anxiety.
2. Trait anxiety.
3. Acute anxiety.
4. Chronic anxiety.

State Anxiety

It is a transitory experience that varies in intensities, fluctuates overtime, tends to occur in relation to an event or situation, anticipated in the near future or present. Occurs in particular situation.

Trait Anxiety

A stable personality characteristic that predisposes people to more frequent and intense anxiety episodes in relation to stress.

Acute Anxiety

An episode of anxiety characterized by intense, symptoms that may occur without apparent warning or accompany a stressful situation in which the person perceives a dilemma to which there is no readily available solution. It occurs for a short period.

Chronic Anxiety

A pervasive, continuous and moderate level of anxiety that has become a part of the personality and is accompanied by chronic insomnia and night mares and episodes of acute anxiety.

Treatment

For mild and moderate anxiety no medical treatment is required. A person should be helped to handle the anxiety situation effectively.

For severe anxiety, anxiolytics are given.

Psychotherapy, behavior therapy are used along with pharmacotherapy

Nursing Management In Acute Stage of Anxiety

1. The person should be removed from the stressful situation.
2. Provide a comfortable position.
3. Record the vital signs.
4. Encourage the person to do diaphragmatic breathing for 5 to 10 min, take long deep breathing for some time.
5. Allow him to verbalize the feeling.
6. Be supportive and give temporary suggestion.
7. Distract the feelings and experience of patient by engaging in positive conversation.
8. If symptoms not controlling, mild anxiolitic drugs can be given.
9. Suggest the person to come for detail work up to do long-term planning.

Nursing Care of Patient with Anxiety Attacks

1. Instruct the clients to keep record of anxiety spells.
   - Arousal of symptoms
   - Intensification
   - Ending
   - Date, time, place, situation
   - Thought, feeling
   - Intervention and its effectiveness
   - Any strategies used and its effectiveness.
2. Instruct the client to analyze has positive and negative expectation of his family, personal, social, and occupational expectation.
3. To examine 'I should and I can't.
4. To follow relaxation technique.
5. To include activities like jogging, walking, swimming, etc in routine life.
6. Teach the importance of verbalizing the problems.
7. Teach them not to fight or argue but change their attitude.
8. Teach assertive techniques.
9. Encourage to attend group meeting of any.
10. To seek for professional assistance when the anxiety interferes in day-to-day life of the person.

Anxiety Disorders

It is recognized that all persons experience anxiety but it is also recognized that some individuals experience such severe anxiety that normally interferes with ability to function in daily life.

There is a general category of anxiety disorders. There are subtypes and six of these are particularly important and common. They are: Generalized anxiety disorders, panic disorders agoraphobia, phobia, obsessive compulsive disorders post-traumatic stress disorder.

Generalized Anxiety Disorder

A generalized anxiety disorder is characterized by unrealistic or excessive anxiety about 2 or more life experiences. It is accompanied by sustained and pervasive feelings of distress and physiologic changes that contribute to the discomfort.

Patient may experience:

- Persistent dread of personal illness some unnamed misfortune be falling them
- Financial failure
- An occupational distresses
- Some unidentified catastrophe.

The anxiety is lasting for 6 weeks and accompanied by:

- Chronic muscular tension
- Restlessness
- Frequent episodes of trembling and shakiness
- Chronic failure and dizziness
- Symptoms of autonomic nervous system hyperactivity—sweating, raised heart rate, cold and clammy skin, etc.
- Vigilance
- Difficulty in concentration
- Sleep disorder (Ans psy Ano 1987)

They usually seek for physical complaints produced by autonomic nervous system hyperactivity, do not come for emotional problem.

Panic Disorder

Panic attacks are unprovoked, sudden episodes of anxiety that usually reach their peak within few minutes and subsides in less than 30 minutes. A sense of dread, which is the most prominent psychological symptom seems to be in reaction to the physical symptoms. They include at least four of a set of specified symptoms. These symptoms include:

Palpitation, or rapid heart rate, sweating, trembling, shortness of breath, sensation of choking, chest pain, nausea, dizziness, fear of losing control, fear of dying, numbness or tingling, chills or hot flushes and some sense of altered reality. They experience fear of dying, loosing their mind, going crazy, unable to control their behavior, sense of impending doom, helpless and being trapped, fear of triggering an episode. They live in constant dread of another attack, hypervigilant, continuously scanning the environment. The tension that becomes a part of the attack. Increases the rest of the attack and vicious circle continues.

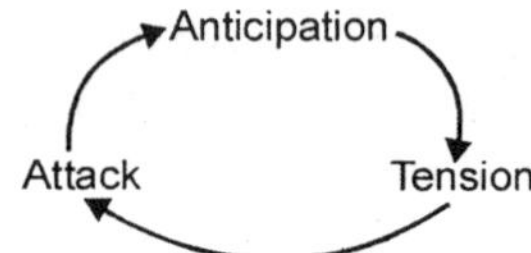

Anticipatory response coupled with the attacks produces pattern of avoidance of places people and situation associated with attacks.

Diagnosis

a. To meet the criteria for panic disorder at least one panic attack must be followed by 1 month or more concern about having one more panic attack.
b. Panic disorder accompanied by agoraphobia

Treatment

Treatment consists of giving:
1. Atidepressant
2. Benzodiazepam
3. Behavior or therapy
4. Psychotherapy

CHAPTER 14

Obsessive Compulsive Disorder (OCD)

INTRODUCTION

Obsessive compulsive disorder is a chronic and distressing disorder that can lead to severe impairment in social academic and family functioning.

It is a common mental illness, earlier it was considered as a rare illness. But studies have now shown that 2 to 3 percent of the population have OCD at some point in their life. Though it is a common illness, and many suffer from the illness, less than 50 percent only have come for treatment. It occurs in all age groups. It is also called the "Doubting disease" 65 percent develops prior to 25 years less than 15 percent develop after the age of 35 years. Data and clinical studies suggest that OCD typically begins during late adolescence or early childhood.

OBSESSIVE COMPULSIVE DISORDER

Definition: According to DSM IV OCD is the presence of obsessions or compulsions that cause marked distress, are timeconsuming and significantly interfere with the persons' normal routine.

Obsessions

These are recurrent or persistent thoughts, impulses, or images that are experienced as intrusive inappropriate, are not simply excess worries about real life problems and that cause marked anxiety or distress.

People feel these thoughts are senseless, irrational, or excessive, but they are unable to control. The thoughts are frightening disgusting and painful, causes significant distress and anxiety or ahead can build to an unbearable level.

Obsessions include fear of germs, fear of harming loved ones, or constant doubt.

Common Obsessions

- Fear of getting dirty, contaminated or infected by people or things in the environment
- Fear of developing a serious life-threatening illness like AIDS, cancer, etc.
- Extreme concern to keep in order, symmetry or exactness
- Fear of committing a crime, such as a theft or harming others
- Recurrent thoughts or images of sexual nature. Fear of thinking exit or sinful thoughts that will go against one's religions
- Fear that some disaster will occur
- Fear of loosing some important things that will be needed later
- Hoarding/collecting obsession
- Extreme concern with certain sound, images, words or number
- Doubts that a task or assignment has been done poorly or incorrectly.

Compulsions

Compulsions are repetitive acts that the person is driven to carryout in spite of knowing that they are meaningless, unnecessary or excessive. These compulsions are meant to reduce their anxiety.

For example, a person may have repetitive thought (obsession) that his hands are contaminated or the stove is not closed, he has to do something to relieve his anxiety so he may wash his hands over and over or check the stove is turned off again and again. These feelings that they must repeat certain actions or rituals are their compulsions.

Very often these rituals/actions to be performed according to certain rules. The retuals may be very simple and hardly noticeable, or they may be very elaborative, sometimes, it will be taking hours to complete and they inference with daily routine. These rituals do lesson the anxiety of the person but only for brief time as fear and tension soon return causing the individual to start the ritual all over again.

Common compulsions are:

- Repeatedly cleaning and grooming behaviors such as washing hands, taking bath, brushing teeth in particular ways.
- Repeatedly cleaning the things in the house.
- Managing things in a certain way touching certain objects in specific way.
- Repeatedly pulling clothes on, then taking them off.
- Counting over and over to a particular number of time.
- Repeating certain action, such as going through a doorway in a specific way or having odd movements while walking.

- Hoarding items such as old electric bills, mail containers, paper, etc.
- Repeatedly checking, locks electrical outlets, gas knobs, light switches, etc.
- Constantly seeking approval.
- Some people with OCD about 25 percent will have only obsessions or compulsions. Most of patient 80 percent will have both obsession and compulsions.

Co-morbidity

Co-morbidity with OCD is common.
The conditions which is associated with OCD are:
- Anxiety disorder
- Depressive disorder
- Behavioral disorder
- Tic disorder.

COURSE OF ILLNESS IN ADULT

For most patient OCD is chronic and lifelong with fluctuation in the severity of symptoms course can be divided in to three categories.
1. Unremitting and chronic.
2. Phasic with periods of complete remission.
3. Episodic with incomplete remission that permitted normal social functioning.
   The course of illness is still under study.

CAUSES OF OCD

Multiple etiological theories are proposed.

Genetic

Fifteen to 20 percent of individuals with OCD come from families in which another immediate family has the same problem. So, most of the researchers believe that there is a biological basis for OCD

Neuropsychiatric

Evidence from neuroimaging, neuro-chemistry and neuropsychology provide substantial support for neuropsychiatric cause. In neuroimaging, the abnormalities in corticostrial, thalamocortical pathways has been identified. PET studies reveals increase glucose metabolism in prefrontal cortex, caudate nucleus, etc.

In biochemical studies serotonin—a neurotransmitter deficiency in the brain is found.

Immunologic

Autoimmune reaction which occurs due to A, B hemolytic streptococcal infection (GABHS). This type is called PANDAS (pediatric autoimmune neuro psychiatric disorder associated with streptococcal infection).

Stress doesn't cause OCD but can precipitate the onset of OCD in a vulnerable individuals strict parenting doesn't cause OCD. Individuals who have been brought up by rigid and strict parents may develop obsessive compulsive personality trait but not OCD.

Treatment

Drug therapy and behavior therapy are mostly used in OCD.

Drug Therapy

SSRIs (Serotonin Reuptake Inhibitors) are given. These drugs increases the amount of serotonin available for nerve cells in the brain. The drugs mostly given are:
- Fluoxietine
- Fluvoxamine

- Sertraline
- Paroxetine
- Citalopram.

Single drug or combination may be used.

The drugs are given for 1 to 2 years or continued for many years.

Behavior Therapy

Is the treatment of choice in OCD Variety of techniques are used to modify the behavior. Exposure and response prevention is widely used which is effective in 60 to 70 percent of people. Principle here is that irrational fears and behavior disappear upon repeated exposure to the source of fear by repeated and prolonged exposure the individuals gets habituated.

Psychotherapy

Supportive psychotherapy is helpful in acute cases and is dealing with obsessive character traits of perfection doubting, procrastination and indecisiveness.

ECT

ECT is also used when the symptoms are un-controlled with drugs and behavior therapy.

Psychosurgery

Is the last choice. It may head to striking reduction in tension and distress cinglectomy may be thought off when symptoms are very problematic.

Nursing problems identified in these patients are:
- Increased anxiety
- Decreased coping ability with compulsion
- Decreased communication

- Ritualistic acts
- Lower self-esteem
- Disturbed sleep
- Need for behavior modification

NURSES ROLE

Primary Prevention

Early treatment brings good results. So early identification is very essentials. Parents and teachers should be educated to identify OCD in early stages.

The OCD symptoms in children will be:

- Poor academic performance
- No concentration
- No happiness
- Depression
- When children have the above problems. The nurse/the teacher/or the parent should discuss in detail for diagnosis and help in getting the treatment
- Public should be made aware that OCD is a mental disorder which needs treatment
- Stress in any area should be avoided or taken care off.

Secondary Prevention

- Importance of medication to control the symptoms to be stressed
- Family to be encouraged to altered educational and support groups
- Encourage patient to engage in behavior therapy
- Family members to be prevented from being part of obsession. Make aware of their role in medication, observation and role in behavior therapy

- Normal activity to be approved
- Provide positive reinforcing techniques when passitive symptoms are observed
- Stress in life should be checked. Unnecessary anxiety should be avoided
- Encourage to maintain personal hygiene at his/her own pace don't hurry him
- Initially allow the patient to continue with his/her ritualistic behavior then set limits but provide adequate time for his rituals
- Direct his mind to other activities which needs concentration
- Teach relaxation technique
- Involve patient in spiritual and recreational activities.

Tertiary Prevention

- Strict follow-up
- Stress management.

BIBLIOGRAPHY

1. Eric Hallarder, and Andrea Allen. The psychiatric clinics of North America. Obsessive-Compulsive spectrum disorder Volume 23 Number 3 September, 2000.

2. Haber, Leach Mc Mahon, Hoiskin, Si Deleau. Comperhensive Psychiatric Nursing, 4th edition. Mosby Year book, 1992.

3. John Andre Allen p.a. centire and Windsey Bergman. Obsessive-Compulsive Disorder of the psychiatric clinics of North America volume 23 Number 3 September, 2000.

CHAPTER 15

Personality Disorders

INTRODUCTION

Personality disorders are developmental conditions, which appear in childhood or adolescence and continue into adulthood. They are not secondary to another mental disorder or brain disease. Personality disorders' are differ from personality changes. Personality changes is acquired during adult life, following severe or prolonged stress, extreme environmental deprivation, serious psychiatric disorder or brain disease or injury.

Personality disorders are subdivided according to cluster of traits or most frequent behavoral manifestation.

Subdivisions of Personality Disorders

Specific personality disorders

    a. Paranoid personality disorder
    b. Schizoid personality disorder
    c. Dissocial personality disorder
    d. Emotionally unstable personality disorder—borderline-impulsive
    e. Histrionic personality disorder
    f. Anankastic personality disorder
    g. Anxious (avoidant) personality disorder

h. Dependent personality disorder
i. Personality disorder unspecified.

Enduring personality changes, not attributable to brain damage and disease

a. Enduring personality changes after catastrophic experience.
b. Enduring personality changes after psychiatric illness.

Habit and impulsive disorders

a. Pathological gambling.
b. Pathological fire setting (pyromania).
c. Pathological stealing (kleptomania).
d. Tricho schiolellomania—pulling the hair to relieve tension.

Gender identify disorder

a. Transexualism
b. Dual role transvertism
c. Gender identity disorder of childhood.

Disorders of sexual preference

a. Fetishism
b. Fetestic transvertism
c. Exhibitionism
d. Voyeurism
e. Pedophilia
f. Sadomasochism
g. Multiple disorder of sexual preference.

Psychological and behavioral disorder associated with sexual development and orientation

a. Sexual maturation disorder.
b. Egodystonic sexual orientation.
c. Sexual relationship disorder.

Other disorders of adult personality

Elaboration of physical symptoms for psychological reasons

Each of the above said personality disorder is diagnosed according to the guidelines given in ICD-10. The personality disorders are conditions comprise deeply ingrained and inducing behavior patterns, manifesting themselves inflexible response to a broad range of personal and social relations.

Each of the above said personality disorder is diagnosed according to the guidelines given in ICD -10. The personality disorders are conditions comprise deeply ingrained and inducing behavior patterns, manifesting themselves inflexible responses to a broad range of personal and social relations. They represent either extreme or significant deviations from the way the average individual in a given culture perceives, thinks, feels and particularly relates to others.

The assessment should be based on as many sources of information as possible. The diagnosis is made only after number of interviews with the individual and with different informants.

The cultural or regional variations in the manifestations of personality conditions are important.

DIAGNOSTIC GUIDELINES OF DISORDERS

Diagnostic guidelines of few disorders of adult personality are given next page.

Paranoid Personality Disorder

This disorder is characterized by:
- Excessive sensitiveness to setbacks and rebuffs
- Tendency to keep grudges persistently
- Recurrent suspicious without justification regarding sexual fidelity of spouse or sexual partner
- A tenacious sense of personal rights out of keeping with the actual situation
- Tendency to experience excessive self-importance, manifest in a persistent self-referential attitude
- Tendency to misinterpret others actions as hostile towards self.

Schizoid Personality Disorder

- Only few activities provide pleasure
- Emotional coldness, detachment or flattened affectivity
- Limited capacity to express either warm, tender feelings or anger towards others
- Apparent indifference to praise or criticism
- Less interest in sexual activities
- Excessive fantasy and introspection
- Lack of close friends and confiding relationship
- Marked insensitivity to prevailing social norms and conventions.

Dissocial Personality Disorder

- Unconcern for the feelings of others
- Gross and persistent attitude of irresponsibility and disregard for social norms, rules and obligation
- Incapacity to maintain enduring relationship though no difficulty to establish them

- Very low tolerance to frustration and low threshold for discharge of aggression
- Incapacity to experience particularly from punishment.

Emotionally Unstable Personality Disorder

- Act without considering the consequences
- Threatening or violent behavior in response to criticism
- Feeling of emptiness
- Unclear, absent self-image, aims, etc.
- Easy to get involved in intense and unstable relationships, later goes to extreme disappointment and even tends for suicide.

Histrionic Personality Disorder

- Self-dramatization, exaggerated expressions of emotions
- Easily influenced by others or circumstances
- Shallow and labile affectivity
- Continuous seeking for excitement when appreciated by others
- Over-concern with physical attractiveness.

Anankastic Personality Disorder

- Feeling of excessive doubt and caution
- Preoccupation with details, rules, tests, orders, organization or schedule.
- Perfectionism that interferes with task completion
- Rigidity and stubbornness
- Unreasonable insistence that other should do everything according to his direction
- Reluctance to allow others to do things
- Insistent and unwelcome thoughts or impulse.

Anxious Personality Disorder

- This personality disorder is characterized by pervasive, persistent feelings of tension and apprehension
- Inferiority
- Excessive preoccupation with being criticized or rejected in social situation
- Restrictions of lifestyle because of need to have physical security
- Avoidance of social or occupational activities that involves significant interpersonal contact because of fear of criticism, disapproval or rejection.

Dependent Personality Disorder

This personality disorder is characterized by:
- Allowing others to make most of one's important life decision
- Subordination of one's own needs to there of others on whom one is dependent
- Unwillingness to make reasonable demands on people one depends on feeling uncomfortable or helpless when alone because of exaggerated fears of inability to care for self
- Limited capacity to make daily decisions without an excessive amount of advise and reassurance from others.

Enduring Personality change after Catastrophic Experience

This disorder is characterized by:
- A holistic or mistrustfull attitude towards the world.
- Social withdrawal
- Feelings of hopelessness and emptiness
- A chronic feeling of being threatened.

Pathological Gambling

It is diagnosed by the guidelines of persistent, repeated gambling, inspite of heavy losses, impaired family relationship and discipline of personal life.

Pathological gambling should be distinguished from gambling and beating, gambling by manic patients.

Pathological Fire Setting

Diagnostic guidelines
- Repeated fire setting without any particular motive, such as monitory gain, or political extremism
- An intense interest in watching fires burn
- Report on feelings of increased tension before setting the fire and intense excitement after the act
- Differential diagnosis should be done from conduct disorder sociopathology schizophrenia, organic psychiatric disorder.

Pathological Stealing (Kleptomania)

- An increased level of tension before the act and experience gratification after the act.
- May feel guilt between the action but will not prevent the repetition.
- Pathological stealing should be distinguished from recurrent shoplifting, organic mental disorder of poor memory and depressive disorder.

Gender Identify Disorder of Childhood is Characterized by

- Perverse and persistent desire to be the opposite sex, to wear the attire (dress) of the opposite sex:

- May be distressed with this thought
- Deny this desire and distress
- More affected in males
- Play with dolls and dress like girls are common in these, boys in the preschool age
- Girls with disorder may be rough
- Interested in sports
- Some of them may continue this and go for homosexuality.

Fetishism

In this disorder some nonliving objects as a stimulants for sexual arousal and sexual gratification. Articles used are human clothings, footwear, rubber/plastic or leather.

Fetishism should be diagnosed only if the fetish is the most important source of sexual gratification. Fetishistic fantasias are not considered as fetishism.

Exhibitionism

It is a condition where a recurrent, persistent tendency to expose the genitals to strangers or to the people in the public places. Commonly this act is followed by masturbation usually happens during stress especially in sexual relationship with desired partners. If the witness appears shacked, frightened or impressed, the exhibitionists excitement is often hightened.

Voyeurism

It is condition in which the individual has persistent recurrent tendancy to look at people engaging in sexual or intimate behavioral such as undressing. This usually leads to sexual excitement and masturbation.

Paedophilia

It is a condition, in which there is a sexual preference for children. Some are interested in girls only some in only boys but others are interested in both girls and boys.

Sadomasochism

In this condition the individual has a preference for sexual activity that involves the infliction of pain or humiliation. The recipient of such stimulation is called masochism and the provider is sadism.

Few other unspecified personality disorders are named in the literature which are not mentioned in this chapter may be either rarely found or found in the combination of other condition, mentioned in this chapter.

MANAGEMENT OF PERSONALITY DISORDER IN ADULTS

The management is done in different steps:

Assessment

Assessment—During assessment it is difficult to make single diagnosis but may be combination of few conditions.

Medical Treatment

Medical treatment—After assessment the medical treatment is given accordingly either by antidepressants, antimanic or antipsychologic drugs.

Psychotherapy

Treatment by dynamic psychotherapy is much the same for personality disorder as for neurosis. It can be carried out individually or in groups. Psychotherapy is not useful in all personality direction. Psychotherapy may help young individuals who lack confidence have difficulty in making relationships and are uncertain about the direction their lives should take. When the psychotherapy is not indicated supervision and support are always useful.

Nursing Management

The nurse should use all psychiatric nursing principles while nursing the individuals with personality disorder. The psychiatric nurse also can be the team member in chemotherapy and psychotherapy also. The treatment for this group of individuals need long-term treatment and supports. The prognosis of disorders of adult personality is not very good.

CHAPTER 16

Mental Retardation or Learning Disability

INTRODUCTION

Mental retardation is a condition in which there is significantly subaverage mental development from birth or early childhood. Most people with mental retardation have the condition from birth. In a small number, the condition may occur following damage to the brain in later childhood. *For example, Brain fever.*

Mental retardation is also termed as mental deficiency, mental subnormality and intellectual deficiency. The words like mental handicap, idiot, imbecile, moron also were used once upon time. As these terms calling stigma, and insult they are not used now-a-days. Recently the term 'Learning disabilities is generally defined in the UK. However, mental retardation is still used in ICD 10 and DSM IV and it is in use in the USA and many other countries.

DEFINITION

Mental retardation is a type of disability marked by impairment or deficiency in general intellectual functioning with onset during developmental years (0-18 years) Most children with MR have the following characteristics:
1. Delayed milestones of development from birth (motor, adaptive, social and language)

2. A slow rate of development compared to normal children leading to a limited intellectual capacity in adulthood.
3. Limited capacity for learning (Satish Chadra Girimaji, 1996)

ICD 10 defined—Mental retardation as a condition of arrested or incomplete development of the mind, which is especially characterized by impairment of skills manifested during development period that contribute to cognitive, language, motor and social abilities.

Generally, it is lifelong condition. Those affected continue to have diminished intellectual capacity throughout their lives. However, in most individuals with mental retardation, those parts of the brain that are not damaged continue to develop. Therefore, they continue to acquire skills and abilities as they grow older adults slowly.

MENTAL RETARDATION AND MENTAL ILLNESS

Mental retardation is not mental illness. The characteristic of mental retardation is delay in mental development, whereas in mental illness, it is disturbance in the mental functions of thinking, feeling and behavior. Mental illness can occur at any age whereas mental retardation is present from childhood. However, mental retardation may also be developmental illness.

Epidemiology

In a survey in the General population in India, it is found that around 2 percent have mental retardation whereas it is estimated about 3 percent among children under 18 years of age. Mild mental retardation is much more common than severe. Mental reardation accounting 65 to 75 percent of all cases with mental retardation.

It has been found that mild mental retardation is more common in rural areas, and in low income groups. It may be due to poor access of health facilities under-stimulation and undernutrition, etc.

Causes of Mental Retardation

Mental retardation results from an impediment to normal brain development. Such an impediment can occur due to variety of reasons.

Mental Retardation may be caused by prenatal, perinatal and postnatal.

Prenatal Causes of Mental Retardation

Genetic disorder

- Chromosomal disorder
- Single gene disorder

Hereditary play a role in some of this disorder.

Chromosomal Disorder

Down syndrome is common cause of mental retardation. Each cell of the body has 46 thread like structures called chromosomes, whereas in Down's syndrome because of a biological error around the time of conception there will be one extra chromosome, i.e 47 chromosomes.

The presence of extra chromosomes interferes with the development of brain causing mental retardation. Children with Down's syndrome will have the charac-terized by:

- Up upstanding eyes, and flat bridge of the nose
- Round face, etc.
- Small mouth and teeth furrowed tongue and high-arched palate, short and broad hands, a curved fifth finger.

Down's syndrome occurs in 1 out of 800 newborn. Though it is a genetic disorder. It is most often not inherited. Can occur in any child. It is more likely to occur in any child. It is more likely to occur when the age of the mother at the time of conception is over 35 years. These children will have good social and interactional skills.

Single Gene Disorder

i. Inherited Metabolic Disorders

The genes in the chromosomes control the growth and maturation of the brain by producing metabolic reactions if these genes are abnormal they may lead to derangement of metabolic reactions and thereby cause mental retardation.

Metabolic Disorder Affect

- Amino acids, *e.g Phynylketonuria.*
- Lipids—Tay-sachs disease.
- Carbohydrates—Galactosemia

ii. Gross Disease of Brain

For example, Tuberose sclerosis. Neurofibromatosis also can cause mental retardation. (Autosomal dominent inheritance)

iii. Brain Malformations

Disease such as genetic microcephalus, hydrocephalus and myelomeningocele can lead to MR.

Other prenatal conditions include
- Deficiencies such as iodine and folic acid in mother
- Severe malnutrition in pregnancy

- Use of substances, such as alcohol, nicotine, and cocaine during early pregnancy
- Exposure to harmful chemicals such as pollutants, heavy metals, use of harmful drugs such as thalidomide, phenytoin and warfarin, etc
- Meternal infections: Rubella and syphill's in 1st trimester can cause MR and visual impairment
- Others–Exposure to radiation and Rh in-compatibility

Perinatal Causes of Mental Retardation

a. Complications of pregnancy
   - Diseases of mother such as heart, kidney and diabetes.
   - Placental dysfunction.

b. Difficult and complicated delivery causing blood supply to the foetus is deprived.
   - Birth trauma
   - Severe prematurity, very low birth weight asphyxia, etc.
   - Neonatal infections like septicemia, jaundice and hypoglycemia.

Postnatal Causes of Mental Retardation

- Brain infections such as tuberculosis, Japanese encephalitis, and bacterial meningitis when they are severe may cause inversible brain damage leading to Mental Retardation (MR).
- Head injury in early childhood
- Chronic lead poisoning
- Severe and prolonged malnutrition
- Gross under stimulation

Causes of Mental Retardation: (Table 16.1)

Table 16.1: Causes of MR

Category	Type	Examples
Prenatal	Chromosomal disorder	Down's syndrome Fragile x syndrome

	Single gene disorder	- Inborn errors of Metabolism *
		  e.g., *Galactosemia*
		- Gross diseases of the brain *
		  phenylketonuria
		- Brain Malformation

	Maternal and environmental influences	- Deficiencies * of iodine
		  folic acid
		- Severe malnutrition
		- Substance abuse *
		- Exposure to harmful chemicals
		- Maternal infection rubella *
		      syphilis *
		- Others – *Radiation exposure
		      * R.H incompatibility

Perinatal	Third trimester
	Labor
	Neonatal first
	4 weeks of life.
		- complications of pregnancy*
		- * Diseases in mother – Heart,
		  kidney and diabetes.
		  Placental dysfunction.
		- severe prematurely, low birth
		  weight, birth asphyxia.
		- Difficult and complicated
		  delivery*
		- Birth trauma*
		- Septicemia, severe jaundice*,
		  hyperglycemia

Postnatal		Brain infection Head injury* Chronic lead exposure* Severe and prolonged mal- nutrition* Gross understimulation*

* Are conditions which can be prevented. (Dr Satish Chandra 1996)

Degrees of Mental Retardation

There are various degrees in mental retardation. The intelligence is measured through a standardized psychological test called IQ test. IQ or intelligence Quotient is a percentage of intelligence a person has in comparison to a normal person from a similar background. An IQ of 100 is normal intelligence. The lesser the IQ the more severe is the level of MR. Based on IQ mental retardation is classified as follows:

IQ	Category
85—100	Normal
70—85	Normal but not retarded
50—69	Mild mental retardation
35—49	Moderate
21—34	Severe
Below 20	profound

Practical way of classifying MR is in two categories. Mild mental retardation with an IQ range of 50 to 70 and severe mental retardation with an IQ below 35.

The table given below shows the attainment of people with different degrees of Mental Retardation in adulthood. It is clear that even a severe MR can be made partly independent in self care skills through proper supervision, care and training.

Degree	1Q range	Adult Attainment
Mild	50-69	Literacy+ Self-help skills ++ Good speech ++ Semi-skilled work +
Moderate	35-49	Literacy +/− Self help skills + Domestic speech+ Unskilled work with or without
Severe	20-34	supervision+ Assisted self-help skills+ Minimum
Profound	Less than 20	speech + Assisted household chores Speech +/- Self-help skill+/−

Note

+ Means attainable.
++ means definitely attainable
+/– means sometimes attainable:
(Taken from WHO Manual Mental Retardation, 1996)

Diagnosis

1. History.
2. Physical examination.
3. Neurological examination.
4. Psychological test (IQ).
5. Laboratory examination—Blood (for Metabolic and enzyme disorder).

COMMON HEALTH PROBLEMS ASSOCIATED WITH MENTAL RETARDATION

Many mentally retarded children and adults are otherwise physically and mentally healthy except they have lower intelligence. Some have other problems. The common problems associated with mental retardation are:

Behavior Problems

Symptoms like restlessness, poor concentration, impulsiveness, temper tantrum, irritability and crying are common. Other disturbing behavior are, aggression, self-injurious behavior (such as head banging) and repetitive racking may also be seen. When they are severe and persistent it becomes lot of stress to the family. So, they should be treated.

Convulsions or Fits

Twenty five percent of mentally retarded will have fit of different kinds. They can be controlled with proper medication.

Sensory Impairment

Difficulties in seeing and hearing are present in about 5 to 10 percent with MR sometimes they can be resolved by hearing aids or glasses or undergoing surgery for cataract.

Other Developmental Disabilities

Disease such as cerebral palsy, speech problems and autism can occur along with mental retardation.

MYTHS AND MISCONCEPTIONS ABOUT MENTAL RETARDATION

Certain Myths and Misconception of MR

1. *Myth:* Mental retardation is hereditary problem.
    Fact: Only a few cases of M.R are hereditary. It is often caused by external influence, some are preventable.
2. *Myth*: Mental retardation is infectious.
    Fact: This is completely false. It cannot be spread by touching or cuddling.
3. Mental retardation is caused by pregnant, and lactating women not following restrictions on food.
    Fact: False. Pregnant and lactating mothers should take good food.
    No food restrictions.
4. Myth tonics/vitamins medicines can cure mental retardation.
    Fact: There is no brain tonics which can stimulate a damaged brain.
    If M.R is caused by a treatable condition appropriate treatment will cure it.
5. *Myth*: Brain operation can cure M.R.

Fact: There are very few conditions leading to M.R which can be cured by surgery.

6. *Myth*: Marriage can cure Mental retardation.
   Fact: This is completely false.

7. *Myth*: Children with M.R become completely normal when they grow up to be adults.
   Fact: Children can make substantial progress as they grow up. But it is unlikely that they will become completely normal.

8. *Myth*: Mentally retarded adults have poor sexual control and bore a danger to others
   Fact: M.R. adults are sexually more inhabited than their normal counterpart.
   Parts.: On the contrary many people become victims of sexual abuse.

9. Mentally retarded cannot be educated or trained
   Fact: It is wrong. Depending upon their degree of M.R, education and training can be given.

10. *Myth*: Faith healers can cure M.R.
    Fact: This is completely untrue.

NURSING CARE OF PATIENT WITH MENTAL RETARDATION

Nursing management consists of:
1. Providing care.
2. Training.
3. Prevention.

Providing Care

Assessment

- Obtain information from the parents regarding what the child can and cannot do

- Find out what the parents would like the child to be trained in, e.g. *Toilet training, speaking abilities, etc.*
- According to the mental age of the child decide on the target activities ranging from the easiest to the more difficult ones.

Psychological Support

- When the parents come to know about the diagnosis they will be in a shock, denial or pain, so console them
- Educate the parents about mental retardation
- Make the parents to accept the child
- Educate the parents about the expected outcome of the child, educate them that there is no complete cure of the disease. They need not seek many doctors finding a solution in this case and spending lot of amount. Instead of that they can save the money so that it will be useful for his future care
- Do not refer the patient to other specialists except, if you suspect any physical condition causing MR, multiple handicaps, or family reaction is not conclusive.

Training

- Training to be given in feeding, dressing, toilet training and social skills such as playing, mixing and interacting with others. Through systemic efforts and using proper technician it is possible to train them in these skills.

BEHAVIOR MODIFICATION TECHNIQUES

These are to be used while modifying the behavior:

Rewarding or Positive Reinforcement

Paying attention, praising the child and giving some material rewards such as sweet, or toys whenever the child shows the desirable behavior or attempts to learn. This will motivate the child to learn new behavior.

Modeling

Showing the child how a particular activity is to be done and encouraging the child to initiate the activity is a powerful method of teaching. Just orally telling or instructing will not help.

Shaping

Shaping means teaching simplified version of a complex activity and gradually making it more and more complex at a pace comfortable to the child.

Chaining

Any activity, e.g. dressing, or toilet training to be broken into several small sequential steps and the child to be taught these skills step by step.

Physical Guidance

When the child cannot learn by modeling, the child can be taught the activity by holding hands and showing them how the work is done. After many such repetitions, the physical guidance can be slowly withdrawn. So, that the child learns to do the task independently.

Modern research has clearly established the utility of these behavioral skills in imparting many kinds of skills.

- There is no age limit for training. It is better to involve normal children with mental retardation children after orienting the normal children.
- Social isolation to be prevented. Group therapy for Mentally retarded adolescents is quite effective.
- Treatment to be given for associative disorder,*e.g. Behavior problem, epilepsy, etc.*

Vocational Training

Vocational training to be given. The jobs can be manual, unskilled or semi-skilled depending on the capabilities of the individual. It is helpful for the mental health, self-satisfaction and social status of these individuals.

Speech Therapy

Mental retardation is often accompanied by a significant limitation in the speech and language development. Systematic application of speech therapy techniques will improve in promotion of speech language and communication.

PREVENTION

Primary prevention

Prevention of occurrence of mental retardation. This includes health promotion and specific protection.

Health promotion
- Health education regarding mental retardation especially in adolescent girls.
- Improving the nutritional status of the community as a whole, especially girls to reduce the risk factors like low birth weight and prematurity.
- Improving pre, peri and postnatal care.

Specific protection
- Universal iodination of salt to prevent iodine deficiency disorder
- Rubella immunization for women before pregnancy
- Administration of folic acid tablets to reduce the occurrence of renal tube defects.
- Nutritional supplementation during pregnancy focusing on intake of calcium and iron.
- Avoiding pregnancy before 21 years of age and after 35 years. The risk of Down's syndrome and other chromosomal disorders increases as the maternal age of pregnancy crosses 35 years.
- Avoiding exposure to harmful chemical and substance including alcohol, nicotine and cocaine during pregnancy.
- Screening pregnant women in infections such as syphilis and promptly treating it.
- Detection and care of high-risk pregnancies.
- Preventing Rh. I SO- 1 minimization a situation which arises when the mother has Rh negative group. This causes damage to fetus which can be prevented by administration of medicine called antidrug. Take immunoglobin immediate after delivery.
- Prompt treatment of severe diarrhea and brain infections during childhood which causes brain damage.
- Universal immunization of children with BCG, Polio, DPT and MMR to prevent many disorder having the possibility to damage brain.
- Preventing chronic low grade exposure to lead
- Genetic counseling.
- Providing an enriching and stimulating environment for children from infancy to ensure proper intellectual development.

Secondary prevention (is halting disease progression)

Secondary prevention consists of early diagnosis and treatment. It can be done by:

- Neonatal screening for treatable disorders like phenylketonuria, galactosemia, and hypothyroidism. Tests are available to detect these disorder at birth itself. These conditions should be detected early and treated.
- Early detection and intervention of developmental delay. Research studies have shown that detecting the mental retardation at an early stage and providing loving and stimulatory environment helps to develop better and prevent many complications (WHO Report, 1996).
- Early detecting and intervention of 'At risk babies' babies born prematurely or with a low birth weight (less than 2kg) or who have suffered birth asphyxia or those who have had a serious illness in the neonatal period to be detected at birth itself and provided good care to prevent mental retardation.

Territory prevention (preventing complications and maximization of functions

In territory prevention disability is limited and rehabilitation is done by:

- Providing proper training in self-help skills which includes care of personal hygiene, grooming, toilet training, communication, etc.
- Training in vocation to be given according to the interest, capability and family resource so that patient can work and spend time in a useful way.
- Family support is very essential. Family encounter different problems at different stages, stress may take many forms, demands of daily care, lack of

leisure time, emotional disturbance, relationship problems within and outside family, etc. are some problems faced by the family.

Parental self-help group

- Organizing/having self-help group for the families of mental retardation will give lot of support to the families and helps in organizing many home based training programs within their community.

TECHNIQUES OF SENSORY MOTOR STIMULATION FOR MENTALLY RETARDED CHILDREN

- Place the child in a sitting position in the mothers lap. Hug the child, rock to and fro, making cooing noise or talking softly to the child
- Tickle the child under the feet, arms and abdomen and elicit laughter from the child
- Place the child sideways in a half reclined position on the mothers lap with legs dangling on side, with one hand supporting the child's head and the other, his abdomen, then rock the child to and fro, the rocking movements have to be accompanied by one particular song/tune with the action
- When the mother is engaged in household activity too, the stimulation of the child can be taken care of by hanging balls and other toys that make sound, hanging colorful cloth pieces of ribbon, balloons, dolls, etc
- Learn to stimulate the child by tickling, stroking, knocking, vocalizing, simple repetitive games, so as to elicit laughter/smile from the child
- Find out several ways of making the child smile like throwing the child up in the air and holding it

- Sit on the chair, keep your legs together and extend forward. Now raise your foot in such a way that the child can be placed at the foot, with his back resting on your legs. Now, raise your legs up and down so that the child is also raised up and down.
- Make use of the available household articles for play such as bangles, key chains, small containers, bells, rubber rings, glasses, spoons, plates, colorful ribbons or cloth pieces, anklets, match boxes, cigarette packs, etc.
- Make use of a torch or a lighted candle light in a slightly darkroom and move if from one end to another; this will help in development of eye movements
- For the child to get various types of experiences the mother or any elder can be made to sit on a swing, placing the child on the lap and playing on the swing, or swing the child sideways holding him/her in you arms
- Cover the child's face with a cloth or hand and remove suddenly saying 'a-ha'
- Give your hands, rattles or other suitable toys to child's hands; let her learn to grasp
- Massage the body with oil; play with her limbs and talk while doing so
- The concept of self and others can be made clear with the help of a mirror. Having the child in front of the mirror and moving away from it, done many times making the child look at herself and the mother, while crying/laughing, in the form of a play, will help the child to identify a baby and an elder in the mirror and later she will identify the reflection as her own.

BIBLIOGRAPHY

1. Mental Retardation team knowledge to action W.H.O Manual, 2001.
2. Dr. Satishchandra Girimaji R. Counselors manual for family intervention in mental Retardation. Indian council of Medical Research Ansarinagar, New Delhi, 1996.

CHAPTER 17

Child and Adolescent
Behavior Problems

INTRODUCTION

The present day is the day of specialization. Psychiatry also not exceptional to this phenomena. Child and Adolescent Psychiatry is special branch of psychiatry as that of gerontology, alcohol and drug abuse so on.

When one carefully observes it can be observed that children and adolescent with abnormal behavior needs special attention. Professionals need to be more observant and patient while handling these group of patients. Children and adolescent may not be expressive to tell their problems. They are to be closely observed before making diagnosis. The behavior modification and the retraining may be more effective for their problems rather medication alone. So, the treating team should have special training, knowledge and aptitude while working in this branch of psychiatry.

The different authors, classify the disorders in children and adolescent in different ways.

CLASSIFICATION OF DISORDERS

In this chapter these disorders are classified as:
   1. Emotional disorder—ED

2. Conduct disorder—CD
3. Attention deficit and hyperkinetic disorder—ADHD
4. Pervasive development disorder—PD
5. Dissociate (coversine) disorder—DD
6. Specific developmental disorder—SDD
7. Schizophrenic disorder
8. Mood disorder
9. Mental retardation.

EMOTIONAL DISORDERS

Emotional disorders are further divided into:
   a. Separation anxiety disorder.
   b. Phobic anxiety disorder.
   c. Social anxiety disorder.
   d. Sibling rivalry disorder.

SEPARATION ANXIETY DISORDER

It is normal in toddlers and preschool children to show anxiety over real or threatened separation from people to whom they are attached.

The key diagnostic features are:
- An unrealistic worry about somebody will leave them and will not return
- Persistent refusal to go to sleep unless the attachment figure is next to them
- Persistent inappropriate fear of being alone.
- Repeated nightmare of separation
- Repeated occurrence of physical symptoms like nausea, vomiting, stomachache when a attached figure is away.

Treatment

Individual counseling: In this method the child is given opportunity to realize the meaning of the problem and also to teach the child some strategies for anxiety management.

Parental counseling: The parents are overprotective counsling. Overanxious make them to realize the problems. Teach them to make the child more independent and allow the child to spend the time with other figures in the family.

Family therapy: After careful assessment if the problem is related to the family system the family counseling is required. Each family member to be explained the nature of the problem and their expected role in the management of the problem.

Drug therapy: Anxolytic drugs are used very rarely in the management of this condition.

Phobic Anxiety Disorder of Childhood

Children like adults can develop fear of different objects and situations. In this type of disorder, there will be persistent, irrational fear of objects, situation or activities. Minor phobic symptoms are common in childhood like animals, insects, darkness death, etc. which are not considered as phobic disorders. They do not exist but gradually disappears as the child grows.

Treatment

Most childhood phobias improve without specific treatment, if that the parents adapt a form and reassuring approach, if it is persisting behavioral modification is the treatment of choice. The different methods of behavioral treatments are:

- Systematic desensitization (gradual introduction of the phobic object or situation while the subject is in a state of relaxation)

- *Flooding*—Which involves persuading the child to remain in the feared situation at maximum intensity and removes the situation gradually. If the phobia is towards school going the term 'school phobia' is used. For school phobia the treatment can involve some special points like
- Involve the parent who has uninvolvement
- Decrease the involvement of the parent who has overinvolvement
- If the child is attending the school with great difficulty take the help from the teacher make the school environment less stressful
- Provide emotional support in the school. If the school attendance is stopped recently, early restart to the school is advisable.

But return to school should be planned well. The school teacher/staff doctor, parents should be involved in planning. Any of emergencies like active anxious behavior of the child should be anticipated and handled properly and firmly.

Social Anxiety Disorder of Childhood

In this disorder show a persistent or recurrent fear and avoidance of strangers. These children are markedly anxious in the presence of strangers and avoid them and this fear interferes with social functioning. Treatment includes simple behavioral techniques and support.

Sibling Rivalry Syndrome

This disorder if characterized by
- The evidence of sibling rivalry and jealousy
- Onset will be followed by the birth of the younger sibling

- Emotional disturbance in a abnormal degree with somatoform disorders
- Attention seeking mechanism
- Physical traumatisation to the sibling
- Bedwetting (Secondary).

Treatment/Management

- Prevention is planned by preparing the child to accept the expected younger sibling in advance
- Try to give appropriate attention to both the children
- Limit setting to the older child
- Help him/her feeling valued
- Make him/her realize the importance his/her role in caring the younger sibling with examples.

NON-ORGANIC ENURESIS

It is a disorder characterized by involuntary voiding of urine by day or night which is abnormal in relation to individuals mental age. And it is not due to lack of bladder control due to any neurological disorder, epileptic attacks or any structural abnormality of urinary tract. Enuresis would not ordinarily be diagnosed in a child under the age of 5 years or with a mental age under 4 years. The enuresis can be primary or secondary. Primary means the child did not attain the bladder control. Secondary means once the child attained bladder control, later due to some emotional stress the child starts enuresis.

Management

- Assessment to exclude the physical pathology:
- Explain the problem to the parents
- Assess the emotional stress and try to reduce it
- Keep a diary to know the pattern of voiding

- Dry nights can be rewarded
- Bladder training is advised
- Belt and pad techniques are used. These techniques are based on the classical conditioning principle. A bell is attached to the napkins, when the child passes urine, alarm starts child has to wake up and change the napkins
- Medication—Antidepressants are used which show considerable improvement.

NON-ORGANIC ENCORPRESIS

It is a voluntary or involuntary passages of feces, usually of normal consistency, in the places not appropriate for that purpose. These are usually associated with emotional disturbances.

Management

- Behavioral techniques to be practiced
- Assess the emotional stress discussing with family members
- Try to reduce the stress and guide the child also to come out of the stress.

FEEDING DISORDERS

Appetite or feeding problems in the children may be symptoms of physical disorders or emotional or relationship problems in the family. Problems may be eating too little, too much, wrong sorts of foods, excessively fussy or choosing to eat or even they starts to eat inedible foods.

ANOREXIA NERVOSA

- It usually occurs in adolescents and young adults.
- It is characterized by:
    Determined food avoidance

A loss or failure to gain weight in the absence of any physical disturbance.

Management

- Assess the emotional problem causing this disorder
- Try to make realize the child the seriousness of problem
- Alter the food habits, plan the diet
- Family should be assessed to see their role causing the problem
- Drug treatment is mainly symptomatic.

Pica of Infancy and Childhood

Pica is the persistent eating of non-nutritive substances such as paper, soil, cloth, etc. It can occur in difficult and undesirable environment, emotional distress, relationship difficulties, autism, mental retardation, nutrition deficiency, etc.

Management

- Look for the cause
- Environmental modification by eliminating the items which are eaten up
- Parental education
- Treat for any type of deficiency.

Stuttering (Stammering)

Speech that is characterized by frequent repetition or prolongation of sounds or syllabus or words by frequent hesitation or pause is called stuttering stammering. It may be due to stress and anxiety, disturbed parent child relationships.

Management

- Assess the stress which cause the condition
- Parents are educated about their role in preventing the condition
- Parents are asked to help the child to pronounce the difficult words
- Child can be referred to speech therapist.

Elective Mutism

It is a condition where there is a persistent refusal to talk in one or more situation, or to individuals despite the abilities to comprehend language and to speak normally in other situation.

Management

It is by stress management which includes individual and family therapy techniques.

Masturbation

This is a disorder where there is a practice of self-manipulation of genitals. At adolescence, masturbation is a universal phenomenon among boys.

Sleep Disorders

a. Nightmares

In this condition unpleasant or frightening dreams occurring during sleep.

Management

- Reduce the anxieties in the day time.
- Do not tell stories of frightening nature
- Control the TV program which can induce fear
- Sedatives can be advised.

b. Sleep Walking–(Somnambulism)

If often occurs in association with nightmares or terrors. The child arises calmly from the bed with blank facial expressions, does not respond to questions. May open the doors goes out, come back safely and close the door and go to bed. When asked in the morning the child may not remember.

Management

- Watch to prevent any untoward incidence during the sleep walking.
- Assess the nightmares if it is accompanied with.
- Manage the nightmares as a part of management of sleep walking.

Thumb Sucking and Nail Biting

Both these behavior are common in children. But when it is persistent and as a part of regression it should be treated.

Management

- Simple instruction or reminder not to do so
- Rewards when it is not done
- Try to find out the underlying problems
- Behavioral therapy at last.

CONDUCT DISORDERS

It is usually defined as persistent antisocial or socially disapproved behavior that often involves damage the property/aggression towards other people and is unresponsive to normal control or authority usually conduct disorders are:

- Excessive levels of fighting

- Cruelty towards animals and people
- Severe destructions of property
- Repeated lying
- Fire setting
- Truancy from school and home
- Temper tantrums
- Persistent disobedience

Treatment

Treatment is mainly to assess and guide the family members to train the child like:

- Enforce the set of rules in the family like rising in the morning, mealtime, study time, etc
- Train the family members to observe the child's behavior and get the touch of his/her feelings
- Ensure consistent supportive behavior, e.g. rewarding the good behavior and bad. Anger management can be taught to the parents
- Individual psychotherapy may be advised
- Group interactions to enforce the peer influence can be implemented
- Antipsychotic drug are used in case of aggressive behavior
- Residential care can be recommended incase if there is compelling reason.

Truancy should be treated separately. Here the management consists of assessment of both home and school situations. Teacher and family members are helped to assess themselves and involve in her treatment by different.

Technique of supporting:
- Understanding
- Modifying
- Accepting

- Adjusting
- Correcting with forms, etc.

Oppositional Defiant Behavior

It is seen under the age of 9 to10 years. It is defined as markedly disobedient, negativistic, hostile, provocative and disruptive behavior which is beyond the normal range of behavior for a child of the same age in the same socio-cultural context.

Management

- Family members are taught to reinforce normal behaviors by praise and rewards and set limits for abnormal behaviors
- Group therapy is recommended by using peer group pressure.

Behavioral Disorder

Attention Deficit + Hyperactivity Disorder (ADHD)

It is characterized by developmentally inappropriate poor attention span or age inappropriate features of hyperactivity and impulsiveness or both. It is 3 times more common among boys. Peeler prevalence is 6 and 9 years, 40 percent children with ADHD has conduct disorders.

The characteristic of ADHD are:

- Impaired attention and overactivity
- Overactivity is accompanied with restlessness, which is not task oriented with disruptive quality
- Premature breaking of tasks
- Impulsiveness
- Over talkativeness with raised tone and pitch.

Management

a. Medical management.

b. *Parental counseling:* Train them how to manage the behavior talking about the possible and treatment.

Introduce to them to difference self-help groups to ventilate problems.

c. Behavioral modification like time out, limit setting, re-enforcing.

d. *Cognitive behavioral techniques:* Teaching behaviors which are more acceptable.

e. Techniques to enhance the attention, e.g. *resorting grain.*

f. Environmental manipulation
   - Intervention at school
   - Placement in small group
   - Time limitation for individual activities
   - Alteration in classroom layout
   - Control of activities or friends at home and school.

Pervasive Developmental Disorder (PDD)

Under this the main disorder is Autism. Autism otherwise known as PDD childhood psychosis, childhood autism pseudo-defective psychosis.

This is characterized by:
- Marked impairment of reciprocal, social and interpersonal interaction
- Social smile-absent
- Lack of awareness of others existence or feelings
- Lack of attachment of parents
- No social play but prefers to be alone
- Marked impairment of making friends
- Lack of limitation
- Absence of fear in the presence of danger
- Lack of verbal or facial response to sound and voices
- Absent and delayed speech
- Echolalia
- Abstract thinking is impaired

- Head banging, body spinning rocking, lining up things
- Symptoms of mental retardation present in 75 percent of autistic children
- Epilepsy is common.

Etiology

Etiology is more of biological, cold apathetic mothers also can cause autism.

Management

Behavior Therapy

- Development of a regular routine with few changes regularly
- Structured class training giving new materials gradually may be planned
- Positive reinforcement is used
- Speech therapy is useful
- Behavior techniques should be used to develop IPR.

Pharmacotherapy

- Fenfluxamine is recommended drug to increase IQ and decrease behavioral symptoms
- Haloperidol decreases the dopamine levels and decrease the hyperactivity
- Other drugs like CPZ, Imipranin multivitamins are given
- Antiepileptics are used in the evidence of seizure attacks
- Psychotherapy to family members to make them to accept and support the child.

Dissociative (Conversion) Disorders (DD)

It is more common in adolescents than in childhood. The word hysteria has been used in so many contexts by psychiatrists.

Common conversion disorders are characterized by:

- Presence of symptoms or deficit effecting motor or sensory function suggesting a medical or neurological disorder. *For example, Dimness of vision, parasthesis, etc.*
- Developmental of symptoms usually in the presence of a significant psychosocial stress.
- Sudden onset
- Patient does not intentionally produce the symptoms
- There may be a secondary gain
- Detailed physical examination and investigation do not reveal any abnormality.

The disorders may affect of motor function, sensory functions, memory, etc.

Management

- Treatment is directed mainly at reducing any stressful circumstances
- Encourage the child to bring out the problem
- Reassurance is needed
- Make the child realize no physical pathology is evident
- Psychotherapy is advised
- Medication is required if child is depressed or anxious
- Try to correct the situation before the child receives the secondary gain.

Somatoform Disorders

In this disorders the child complain of somatic symptom where there is no pathology is evident. Common complains may be abdominal pain, headache and leg pain.

Management

Management may be of dissociate disorder.

SDD (Specific Development Disorder)

Under developmental disorders specific developmental disorders specially learning disorders are getting much attention. They are known under the heading of Specific Learning Disorders (SLD) common learning disorders are:

- Reading backwardness
- Reading retardation
- Difficulty in learning spelling
- Difficulty in arithmetic addition
- Difficulty or retardation in writing.

Reading Backwardness

In this the child's reading ability is poor in relation to the average children of the same age regardless the intelligence:

Reading Retardation

In this the achievement is low after taking both age and intelligence into account is that there is a specific educational disability.

General reading backwardness and retardation affect the children in their other learning abilities. Over neurological problems or developmental delays, such as dysprasia are common among them. These children are mainly from large families or low socioeconomic classes.

Specific retardation is usually associated with some over neurological problems and it is running in families.

Difficulty in Learning Spelling

This may be in association to reading backwardness and retardation. In this condition child is not able to remember the spelling of words. It can be jumbling of spelling, e.g.: instead of 'gelpen' the child writes 'genpel'. It can happen in reading also instead of reading 'reading' the child may read 'leading'.

In certain children they hardly remember the spelling, so never can complete the word, by missing an alphabet in the word. Many a time an alphabet can change the word, word makes a different meaning and the whole answer may go wrong. This group of children may be good in personal interviews and practical examinations. But poor in written examination.

The Other Group go for Developmental Dysphases

It is a condition in which with normal intelligence and language stimuli, the child is slow to develop language. Once the language is developed the articulation may become a problem. These children may be good in written examinations but may not fair in personal interviews. The world used for this condition is so confusing they are: dyslexia, word blindness, specific reading or talking disability.

All the above said problems may be associated with antisocial behavior. Emotional disorder may also exist in reading or spelling disorders.

Management

- Assessment of physical problems which contribute for speech and language problem and treat them in a possible way.
- Psychological assessment is necessary to put them into the groups where they fit into, while giving training to them.
- Individually tailored training is given.
- Parents are counseled to make them aware of their role in the management.
- Parents are given knowledge and skill to handle these children.
- Can be sent to special schools if available.

SCHIZOPHRENIA

Children are rarely affected but reported. The sign and symptoms and manifestation are same as in schizophrenia in adults. Child may be withdrawn for sometime and may start in inappropriate affect and later develop hallucination and delusions of various types.

Management
- Antipsychotic drugs
- Provide specialized schools if possible
- Parental counseling is necessary.

MOOD DISORDERS (MD)

Mood disorders in children and adolescents have received increasing recognition and attention over past few years. Depressive disorders make the child irritated, loss of interest in eating , sleeping. It can show the symptoms of lethargy diminished ability to work study think and concentrate. Even the child can go to commit suicide.

Management

- Drug management is necessary (Antidepressants)
- Social skill training
- Psychotherapy
- Family education, etc.

MENTAL RETARDATION

Mental retardation is dealt in a separate chapter of this book.

NURSES ROLE IN CHILDREN AND ADOLESCENT PSYCHIATRY

- As it is happening in any branch of nursing, the nurse should get special training before posted to children and adolescent psychiatry
- The nurse should have the knowledge of etiology of these problems
- They should be observant to get the history to make diagnosis as early as possible
- As many of these conditions are treated in behavioral modifications the nurse should have the experience and training to handle these children
- The nurses should be able to assess the parents behavior which can contribute or trigger the behavioral problems of the child
- The nurse should be able to correct and guide the parents in day today activities while they are in hospital. This therapeutic communication and skills should be helping them to manage the children at home
- The nurse should be supportive for the family members

- The nurse should take care of drug therapy whenever is necessary
- The nurse should conduct group therapies, play therapies, etc. in collaboration with other team members
- The most important role of nurse in this area is to prevent such disorders in other children of the family unless it is genetic
- If genetic, genetic counseling is to be recommended to the parents.

BIBLIOGRAPHY

1. Essentials of Child psychiatry. HM Connell Blackwell publication, 1985.

CHAPTER **18**

Geriatric Nursing

INTRODUCTION

Nursing for elderly is otherwise known as geriatric nursing. The word geriatric came from two words 1. *geros*-aging and *iatric*-detoriation. Any living being grow old and its ability in different function detoriates. Present day aging and its problems attracted the medical and paramedical professionals. So, nursing also finds its special branch to care this population.

Why geriatric care is special? It is because the population is vulnerable to different type of problems which need special attention. This attention can be preventive, curative and promotive.

When does aging starts? There are so many studies and findings in this regard. But all of them differ in their findings. There are eminent people who felt that detoriation starts from the birth itself. It may not be true when one looks at the actual growth of a child to adulthood. Generally, the symptoms of aging starts after the age of 50 and it affects the normal functioning of an individual by the age of 58 to 60. It may be the reason the retiring age for the employed group is 58 to 60.

Though the symptoms of aging are evident after 50, the change in the anatomy and physiology starts from the age of 35 to 40.

When aging occurs at a expected age at expected rate it is considered normal aging. There are cases where there is evidence of aging at an early age and at a speedy rate, then it is called pathological aging.

Normal aging caused by the natures law. Any living organisms die after certain period. The period between birth and death is always a period of detoriation. It can be applied to a plant, animal and in human being also. The normal aging in human being occurs because of the following reasons:

Changes in Anatomy

To certain extent repair and regeneration taken place in every organ of the body part. Later the ability for repair and regeneration or not adequate and each system of the body becomes weak in its functions.

For example, heart not able to pump the blood effectively. Since blood circulation to each tissue is important for its nutrition, when blood, circulation is not sufficient it starts detoriation in its functioning.

Changes in Physiology

For every activity in the different systems of the body depends upon the normal physiology, for the normal physiology every organ needs good blood circulation. When there is decrease in blood supply to the brain the mental ability detoriates. The diminition in gastric juices will cause decrease in appetite, decreases in digestion. This will indirectly affects the general ability in both physically and mentally.

Neurochemical Changes

Normal tear and wear in the neurons may cause the imbalance in the neurochemical mechanism plays a an important role in normal behavior. So, change in this system will cause the inability in controlling the emotion. Which can cause other behavior problems which needs intervention.

Pathological Causes

The hypotrophy or hypertrophy of different organs can cause detoriation of normal functions in an individual. Hypertrophy of prostrate gland in man cause in difficulty in voiding finally retention and overflow. Hypotrophy in the vagina in females can cause incontinence. Hypertrophy of brain tissue can cause changes in mental ability. An enlargement of ventricles of the brain causes memory deficit, ataxia and so on.

Social Changes

This may be in the family, where children are away because of studies, job or got married. This is the time of retirement where they loose the close friends. Death of the spouse is another reason where the individual can detorate. The modernization of the world may make these individuals cannot utilize the facilities and they may become depressed and withdrawn from the society. Place for living also may become a problem for elderly.

PROBLEMS EXPECTED IN ELDERLY

Due to the gradual detoriation in the body organs the individual experience problems in every system of the body.

1. *Alimentary system*: Decreased appetite, inability to digest, inability to take good quantity of food, inability to digest certain high caloric food.
2. *Respiratory system and circulating system*: High blood pressure, cerebrovascular accidents, anemia are the common problems.

3. *Urinary system*: Frequency of micturation, retention with overflow, repeated urinary infection.
4. *Musculoskeletal system*: Slow in motion, arthritis osteoarthritis.
5. *Sensory organs*: Loss of hearing, dried skin, changes in vision, inability to enjoy the taste of food.
6. *Nervous system*: Detoriation in memory, inability to judge, inability to control emotions.

Though many of these repeated problems are mentioned here many unexpected and related problems which are not listed here.

GERIATRY AND PSYCHIATRY

More than any branch of medicine psychiatry is preparing its professional to care this population, because all physical problems when it is not cured with medicines these individuals exhibit many behavioral problems.

The reasons for behavioral problems are:

1. *Changes in the physical appearance*: It can make the individual depressed. The changes may be in structure, like weight, dropping shoulder, balding, greying, dryness of skins discoloration of skin, etc.
2. *Changes in the physical mobility*: The movement may become slow and restricted for these people which can make them depressed or irritated.
3. *Changes in finance*: Once they become retired the money flow is lets or they may have to depend on their children. Many are not prepared for this stage so they become depressed or agitated, or even go for wandering.
4. *Problems related to food*: Since they cannot eat properly, they get irritated fast, when the appetite is not good they blame others for not cooking properly. This make them physically weak because of poor nutrition.

5. *Problems related to the loss of dear ones*: It may be the death of the spouse. Some of them experience the separation of children. Grief reaction may be so severe, where intervention is necessary.

Management

Management is to directed more preventive than treatment. Treatment by medication is advised when it is necessary. Nursing management should have three dimensions.
1. Prevention.
2. Treatment with medication.
3. Rehabilitation to prevent further detoriation.

Prevention

Prevention of aging is a myth. But prevention of behavioral changes in an individual due to aging can be prevented to certain extent. How it is possible. It is mainly by making the people aware of the expected problems in life at different stages. Give the suggestions which can be practical to each individual. Guide them to choose the method every now and then.
The guidelines for preventing the problems in old age
1. Balanced diet.
2. Good exercise to keep the body fit.
3. Plan well the finance periodically.
4. Health checkup after the 35 years.
5. Prepare to accept the separation of children by marriage, job or study.
6. Prepare to accept the death of the spouse and plan where to live after.
7. Become member of any club to evenings if affordable.

Treatment

Once the problems occur they are managed by:

a. *Drugs*: If needed to treat depression or manic symptoms

b. *Diet*: Small meals, with low protein and fat can be advised. Vitamins should be supplemented. If oral food is not possible, Ryles tube feed is recommended.

c. *Building*: The building where they live can be modified with wide doors, comfortable commode in toilet, good lighting every room electric switches can be near the bed, calling bells can be provided to use in case of emergency.

d. *Recreation*: Facilities for recreation can be provided according to the condition of the individual. It can be Television, if the sight is good, a radio can be given to a person when hearing is good, indoor games can be allowed and facilitated for a person who can walk and come to a common room, outdoor games can be recommended for a person who can do so.

e. *Social visits*: It can be planned either taking them out or allowing other groups to visit them.

f. *Spiritual need*: It should be met according to their faith.

g. *Rehabilitation*: It can be in different ways. They can be given some useful work according to their ability. The money which is earned may be utilized for them. These rehabilitation may be only for spending the time usefully and effectively. It also may be to keep the mental abilities opt.

h. *Exercise*: Exercise can be active or passive.

i. *Communication*: Detoriation in vision and hearing may make the communication difficult. So, hearing aid or sight glasses can be provided. Writing pad and pen can be provided for communication, calling bell can be useful. Models and charts can be given to indicate the needs.

   j. *Bladder and bowel*: Special care to this individuals is necessary. As females are more prone to urinary infection teach them the necessity of cleaning after each time of voidance. Constipation to be treated with food with good roughage, plenty of fluids, etc.

   k. *Residence*: Nursing homes can be planned for individual which can solve not only the problems of shelter but the problem socialization, there they have inmates who can act as self-help group. Group of same age and some problems can make them happy and enjoy the life. Sharing their experience, may also learn how to face their challenges looking at other's problems.

Geriatric problems is a problem of today and tomorrow. So, a good planning and action to prevent the problems of aging population is the challenge of today. Planning out the national level is recommended in this regard.

CHAPTER 19

Alcohol and Drug Abuse

INTRODUCTION

Alcohol and drug abuse is the common term used in many literature. But instead of drug, substance is the best word because they are not always drugs which are used for therapeutic use.

Why people use an abuse alcohol or substance? It may be:

- To have pleasurable effect.
- To avoid or lessen the unpleasant effect (physical or psychological trauma).
- Increase the amount of substance to get some effect (Due to tolerance the same amount may not give same effect as before)

When do you call it is an abuse?

Before making a diagnosis it is important to know that:

- How frequent the individual abuses?
- What is the amount of intake?
- What is taken or abused?
- How long the substance is being taken?
- What are the associated problems that is physical problem?
- Psychological problems

- Problems in IPR (Interpersonal Relationship)
- Problems in family: occupation and society etc.,

The common terms used while dealing with alcohol and substa nce abuse are:

DRUG

Drug is a medicinal product, any substance in a pharmaceutical product that is used to modify or explore physiological systems or pathological status for the benefit of receiptants. This term is also used to refer to substances of abuse among which some people include alcohol, tobacco, caffeine, etc.—WHO (1989).

DRUG ABUSE

It refers to the persistent or sporadic excessive use of a drug, inconsistent with or unrelated to acceptable medical practice—WHO 1969.

Tolerance and Crosstolerance are Generally Understood in Pharmacology

As a decrease in response to drug dose that occurs with continued use and the development of tolerance to another substance, which the individual has not previously been exposed to as a result of acute or chronic intake of substance respectively.

Dependency

It can be psychological or physical, or both.

Psychological Dependency

It is a condition in which a drug produces a feeling of satisfactory and or psychic drive that require periodic or continuous administration of the drug to produce pleasure or to avoid discomfort (1974).

Physical Dependency

It is an adoptive state that manifests itself by intense physical disturbances in the withdrawal or abstinence syndromes, which made-up of specific arrays of symptoms and signs of psychic and physical nature that are characteristic for each drug type (WHO 1974).

Withdrawal Symptoms

These are psychological and physiological reactions to the reduction or complete withdrawal of the substance of use. How long withdrawal symptoms lasts, often depends upon the previous use of substances and on the nature and extends of both physiological and psychological dependence (Cooper 1994).

Acute Intoxication

A transient condition following the administration of the alcohol or other psychoactive substance, resulting in disturbances in level of consciousness, cognitive, perception affect/behavior or other psychophysical functions and responses (ICD 10).

Withdrawal State

A group of symptoms of variable clustering and severity occurring on absolute or relative withdrawal of substance after repeated and usually prolonged and high dose, use of that substance.

Withdrawal State With Delirium

A state in which the withdrawal symptoms are complicated with delirium.

Delirium Tremors

It is short lived but life threatening, toxic confusional state with somatic disturbances. It is usually a consequence of partial or complete withdrawal of alcohol in individual who has history of usage of alcohol for a long years.

Psychotic Disorders in Alcohol and Substance Abuse

It is a cluster of psychotic phenomena that occur during or immediately after psychoactive substance use and are characterized by hallucinations, delusions ideas of reference, psychomotor disturbances, abnormal affect.

The major dependence producing drug are:

1. Tobacco.
2. Alcohol.
3. Opiates.
4. Cocaine.
5. Sedatives and hypnotics.
6. Amphetamine.
7. Inhalants—volatile solvents.
8. Hallucinogens.

Etiology of Substance Abuse

1. Psychological factors: It is seen in personality disorders only with curiosity to experience the effect.
2. Biologic factors.
   - Genetic factors.
   - Biochemical factors.
3. Social factors.
   Peer pressure, easy availability, poor social family support, permissive social attitude, etc.

Alcohol Abuse and Management

Many societies accept the use of ethyl alcohol as a psychotropic drug for adults. It also played an important role in the development of human civilization for last many centuries. It has been used as medicine, in religious ceremonies and as a drink to enhance the social interactions.

Alcohol consists of carbon, hydrogen and oxygen. For stronger effect distillation is required.

Patterns of Consumption

Starts with social drinking only evenings and night
- When get tired
- When get tensed
- When alone
- Increase the frequency
- Increase the quantity because of tolerance
- Start drinking anytime of the day
- No life without drink
- Withdrawal symptoms if does not drink.

CONSEQUENCES OR PROBLEMS OF EXCESSIVE USE OF ALCOHOL

Physical Problems

- **G.I Tract**
- Acute gastritis, gastric ulcers, fatty liver, cirrhosis of liver, esophagitis, esophagal varies, peptic ulcer, cancer of liver or stomach, pancreatit's.
- **CNS**
- Hallucination, delusions, alcohol jealousy, peripheral neuropathy, amnesia, dementia, suicidal tendency, delirium, tremors, ataxia.

Miscellaneous

Anaemia, malnutrition, sexual disfunction.

Social Problems

- Marital disharmony
- Financial crisis
- Occupational hazards (interest, loss of jobs).
- Incidence of other drug abuse
- Accident during driving, or using machineries
- Legal problems like driving while drunk, theft to get money to buy the alcohol.

Management

During Acute Intoxication

If the individual in intoxicated stage is brought to casualty.

- Draw the blood for all routine investigations including biochemical, renal function, liver function, SGPT, SGOT, etc.
- Give I/V fluids to remove the toxic effect
- Infuse multivitamin
- Sedate if necessary like confusion manic or abusive behavior
- Once the acute stage is over
- Take the history of nature, amount and any other drug is abused
- Admit the patient for therapy
- If motivated drugs for deaddiction can be started
- If not motivated individual therapy, group therapy can be given
- Nursing management for all symptoms should be planned and implemented
- Family should be interviewed, guided, for future management.

Opiates Abuse and Management

Opiates are otherwise known as narcotic analgesics. They are derived from the plant poppy. They and their synthetic preparation are known as opiates. Some of the opiates preparation are:

Natural Alkaloids

- Morphine
- Codeine

Some Synthetic Preparation

- Heroin, Brown sugar

Pure Synthetic Preparation

- Pethadine
- Tridegesic

Complications

The effect depends upon the route and form of usage. If the drugs are taken intravenously the effect is fast but less intense. If moderately used they depress CNS, dilating the blood vessels, leads constipation. At higher doses the person becomes sedated and drowsy. With higher dose, stupor, coma, death associated with respiratory failure is expected. Withdrawal symptoms occur as early as a few hours after the last administration.

Management

- Try to keep them away from source
- Individual psychotherapy
- Group therapy

- Family counseling to identify the cause and remove them.

Cocaine Abuse and Management

It is powerful short lasting CNS stimulant and local anesthetic. It is derived from *ERYTHROXYLON COCA* and *ERYTHROXYLON* species in South America.

Modes of Abuse

- Chewing the leaves
- Keeping it between cheek and teeth, sniffing
- Injection
- Smoking.

Complication: When abused.

- Malnutrition, decreased sleep agitation. Bouts of paranoia, confusion, mood swings. Repeated sniffing damages the nasal mucosa.

Management

- Psychotherapy
- Group therapy

Family involved program to find out the basic cause and treat them.

Sedative and Hypnotics Abuse and Management

The common substance used are:
- Barbiturates of different strength and Benzo-diazepines, etc.

These are the drugs used for therapeutics effect. Later the individuals become addicted and later dependant.

Intoxication and Effects

Intoxication and effects depends upon the drug used or dosage used. It varies from simple sedation to death. It may go through various degree of effects like:

- Increased sleeping pattern
- Irritability
- Increased speech
- Swinging of mood
- Slurring of speech
- Memory impairment
- Diplopia
- Nystagmus
- Respiratory depression
- Coma
- Death.

Complication

- Damage to liver
- Damage to kidney
- Respiratory depression
- Convulsions
- Coma, death
- Other legal complication
- Like illegal driving
- Stealing, etc.

Inhalants and Volatile Solvent

Commonly used volatile solvents

- Petrol
- Glues
- Spray paints
- Varnish
- Varnish remover
- Industrial solvents.

Intoxication Effects

- Euphoria
- Excitement
- Dizziness
- Slurring of speech
- Apathy
- Impaired judgment
- CNS complication including respiratory insufficiency and death.

Complication

Its complications are as follows:
- Irreversible damage to liver and kidney
- Peripheral neuropathy
- Perceptual disturbances
- Brain damage
- Personality disorder
- Activity.

Management

- Avoid the easy accessibility of abused substance
- Personal guidance
- Group therapy
- Family involving therapies
- Find out the root cause of this behavior and treat them.

Hallucinogens Abuse and Management

Hallucinogens are otherwise called psycheodelics and psychotogenes. The key difference from other classes of drugs is their ability to alter perceptual function.

The substance used are:
- L.SD (Lysergic acid diethlamide)

- Hallucinogenic mushrooms
- Cannabis

1. Lysergic Acid Diethlamide (LSD)

It is a white powder derived from *Ergot*, a fungus found growing on grasses. It is very powerful and potent, only few micrograms are required for effect. In later half of 20th century LSD was used to assist in recovery of unconscious and repressed thoughts and feelings during psychotherapy. Later its therapeutics use was decreased. And started using by people who want mystical experiences including a sense of increased creativity and search for new meaning to things around them.

It is used as tablets mixed with some other drugs. It is available in solution form, then it is used on gelatin, sugar cubes, etc.

Effect and Intoxication

Effect starts within 30 minutes of ingestion and can last for several hours. The effect also depend up on the dosage taken.

Once the effect starts the individual will feel.

- Excitement
- Agitation
- Perception disorder including intensified colors, distorted shapes, sizes, movement in stationary objects
- Dizziness
- Increased blood pressure
- Dilation of pupil
- Relaxation of long muscle
- Making the person flaccid.

Management

- Try to avoid the easy availability of the substance.
- Individual psychotherapy
- Group therapy
- Family involvement to see the root cause and treat them.

Hallucinogenic Mushroom Abuse and Management

- A great variety of hallucinogenic plant were used by ancient civilisation. It is reported to have 100 varieties of such plants available all over the world. The consumption is by eating. Effect is like mild LSD. It may be causing:
- Euphoria,
- Perception distortion

If the mushroom is poisonus when eaten death can occur.

Use of Cannabis and Management

Cannabis is derived from cannabis sativa, a green bushy plant. The cannabis is used in different form, like dried material which is known as marijuana, ganja. This is dried form the different part of the plants like leaf, flower, etc.

Use of Cannabis

Individuals use cannabis in different forms like in the form of:
- Plant
- Leave
- Charas
- Bang

- Ganja—Marijuana etc, Some of them are mild but when abused, gives all the effects like intoxication, dependency and withdrawal symptoms.

Complication

Its complications are as follows:
- Transient—short lasting—psychiatric disorder
- Amotivation like lethargy, laziness, absenting from work or studies.
- Other complication like, memory impairment, mood disorder, use of other psychoactive drugs, stealing, pulmonary diseases.

Management

- Hospitalization
- Individual therapy
- Group therapy
- Family therapy
  Supportive measures to occupy himself to get away from habits.

NURSES RESPONSIBILITIES IN ALCOHOL AND SUBSTANCE ABUSE

For each substance and alcohol abuse the management is mentioned separately in this chapter. But in general nurses have some responsibilities in the management of substance and alcohol abuse.

It can be discussed under:
1. Prevention of occurring.
2. Management of acute stage.
3. Management in transient stage.
4. Prevention of relapse.

Prevention of Occurring

This prevention can be done by:

School health nurse: School health nurse during her routine health checkup and interviews can identify the stress among individual children who can go for abuse of alcohol and substances. She needs to counsel the children individually and parents if needed. She also can give health talks to children from time to time to get away from bad habits.

Community nurse: Community nurse can identify the group who is involved in abusing substance and alcohol. She also can warn and divert the group who are susceptible for abuse. She also can identify the easy available resources of these substances. And with the help of leaders and governmental policies these resources can be banned especially for beginners.

Mental health nurse: Mental health nurse should use of her ability to build healthier families and communities. A healthy family and community can prevent the stresses. The reduction in stress in families and healthy community will definitely prevent the substance and drug abuse.

Nurse in general hospitals: The nurse in general hospitals are expected to do holistic nursing. While nursing an individual holistically the nurse can find out the possibilities of individuals going to the habit of using alcohol and drug to reduce the physical pain or to get away from unpleasant situation. The nurse can anticipate these and guide them different methods to prevent these habits.

Nursing Management During the Acute Stage of Alcohol and Drug Abuse

The nurse should be taking the following steps during the acute stage who comes in intoxication:
- Draw the blood for blood investigations including routine, liver function, renal functions electrolytes and HIV
- Hydrate and remove the toxins
- Supplement with vitamins
- Give sedation if the individual is abusive and assaultive.
- Watch for any suicidal and homicidal behavior
- Keep the individual in inpatient care till the general health improves.

Nursing Management of Transient Stages

In this stage the nurse can give individual therapy to motivate the individual. She can use her psychiatric nursing principles to get the confidence. This motivation should help him to under go deaddiction therapy. And this should also help the individual to have the strength to be abstinent.

Nursing Responsibility to Prevent Relapse

Individual therapies and family therapy should be used to prevent relapse. Many times not only the individual is responsible for abuse of alcohol or drug. The family members do play an important role to make these individual substance or alcohol dependent.

So along with all professionals in medical and paramedical the nurses also do play very important role in prevention and management of alcohol and substance abuse.

BIBLIOGRAPHY

1. James Kennedy and Jean F anger Drug and alcohol dependences nursing Human Nsg- 1987
2. ICD - 10

CHAPTER 20

Organic Mental Disorders

INTRODUCTION

Organic mental disorders are disorders which have a demonstrable and independently diagnosable cerebral disease or disorder. In simple way, organic mental disorders are disorder which have an organic cause.

Some organic brain illness can mimic any psychiatric disorder, especially in the initial stages. So in evaluating a patient with any psychological or behavioral problems organic cause should be given the first consideration.

ORGANIC MENTAL DISORDER

Organic Mental Disorder may occur due to:
1. Demonstrable structural diseases of the brain, e.g. Brain tumors, injuries, degeneration, etc.
2. Brain dysfunction caused by diseases outside the brain, e.g. Myxedema, epilepsy.
3. Sleep disorders (are included in organic mental disorders).

Organic Mental Disorder should be suspected when patients have:
1. First episode.
2. Sudden onset.

3. Old age.
4. History of alcohol and drug abuse.
5. History of any injury, epilepsy or loss of consciousness.
6. Presence of confusion and disorientation.
7. Hallucination of different types.

Classification

1. Organic disorders are classified according to the psychological impairment whether it is generalize or specific. Generalized impairment affects cognition, mood and behavior. Specific impairment affect one or two function, memory, thinking or mood.
2. It also can be classified whether the syndrome is acute or chronic.
3. Whether the underlying dysfunctions of the brain generalized or focal. Generalized dysfunction can come from tumors in the temporal lobe, etc.

So, the diseases can be classified into the four conditions.

a. Delirium.
b. Dementia.
c. Amnesic syndrome.
d. Other organic mental disorders.

DELIRIUM

This is also called acute organic psychiatric syndrome. Delirium is the commonest organic disorder characterized by impairment of consciousness. Five to fifteen percent of all patients in medical and surgical wards and 20 to 30 percent of patients in surgical intensive care units will have delirium (Lipowski 1980) most cases recover quickly only a few are seen by psychiatrist.

Clinical Features

1. Acute onset
2. Impairment of consciousness, characterized by slowness, poor concentration decreased awareness to surroundings, disorientation to time, clouding of consciousness, decreased attention span etc.
3. Marked perceptual disorder.
   a. For example, illusions misinterpretation and visual hallucination.
4. Disturbance of sleep wake cycle most commonly insomnia at night and daytime drowsiness.
5. Thinking is slow and muddled ideas of reference and delusions are common but transient.
6. Emotional disturbances such as anxiety, depression or lability are common.
7. Disorientation in time and pacing as invariable and important features.
8. Disturbance of memory affects registration, retention and recall.
9. Insight impaired.

Causes of Delirium (Acute Organic Syndrome)

The causes are:
- Drug intoxication
- Withdrawal of alcohol and drug
- Metabolic failures, e.g. uremia liver failure, etc.
- Endocrine disorders
- Systemic infections
- Intracranial infection
- Other intra-cranial causes
- Head injury
- Nutritional deficiencies
- Epilepsy.

Diagnosis is done mainly by clinical symptoms, no laboratory test is diagnostic but it will help in finding the etiology:

1. Management consists of identification of cause and immediate correction.
2. Symptomatic measures like benzodiazepines (diazepam 10 mg) or antipsychotics (haloperidol /5 gm) may be given and maintenance treatment with oral haloperidol till recovery occurs.
3. Supportive medical and nursing care given appropriately.

Nursing Care

Nursing care for patients with acute organic disorder consists of:

- Providing safe and protected environment for the patients to protect himself and to protect others. So there should be:
    - Less stimuli around him
    - Disturbing items should not be in the room
    - Clam and well-illuminated room
    - Continuous supervision.
- Reduce patient's fear and anxiety.
    - Avoid misinterpreting subjects and objects.
    - Allow him to ventilate his fears and support.
- Meet the physical needs.
- Reorient to the place and person now and then.
- Resocialize and provide other symptomatic nursing measures.

DEMENTIA (CHRONIC ORGANIC PSYCHIATRIC SYNDROME)

Dementia is generalized impairment of intelligences, memory and personality without impairment of consciousness.

The impairment of all functions occur globally causing interference with day to day activities and interpersonal relationship. It is an acquired disorder and most of the cases are irreversible a small but important group are remediable.

Clinical Manifestation

1. Impairment of memory (predominantly of recent memory).
2. Changes in personality.
3. Impairment of judgment and impulse control.
4. Emotional lability.
5. Thought abnormality slow thinking, persecutory delusion.
6. Disorientation in time, place, person.
7. Urinary and fecal incontinence may develop in later stages.

The cause of Dementia are:
- Degenerative conditions like
    - Senile dementia
    - Alzeimer's disease
    - Picks disease
    - Huntington's chorea
    - Parkingson's disease
    - Multiple sclerosis
    - Normal pressure hydrocephalus.
- Intracranial space occupying lesions
    - Tumors, subdural hematomas
- Traumatic
    - Head injuries
- Infection
    - Encephalitis of any cause, neurosyphilis
- Vascular
    - Multi-infarct dementia occlusions and arteries

- Metabolic
    - Uremia, liver failure, etc.
- Toxic
    - Alcohol, poison
    - Anoxia
    - Anemia, postanesthesia
- Vitamin deficiency
    - Sustained lack of B_{12}.

Treatment

It consists of:
1. Basic investigation.
2. Treating the underlying cause if treatable.
3. Symptomatic management.
   a. Environmental manipulation to reduce stress.
   b. Treatment of medical complication.
   c. Treating anxiety with benzodiazepines.
   d. Low doses of antipsychotics for psychiatric symptoms.
   e. Short-term hospitalization.
   f. Institutionalisation may be necessary in later stages.
   g. Specific drug treatment, e.g. Donepezil or Rivastigmine in Alzheimer's diseases.

Nursing Management

1. *Assessment*

   Careful and meticulous assessment of patient is very important before planning the nursing care.
   - Observe and analyze patient's abilities to perform ADL (Activities of Daily Living), eating, bathing dressing, etc.
   - Involve family members in planning and care.

2. *Maintaining peak physical health*

One of the most essential nursing action is to facilitate optional functioning by maintaining physical health.
- Eye glasses for poor vision
- Hearing aids for diminished hearing
- Any other physical problem to be taken care of.

3. *Structuring the environment*

According to need and sensory level
- Provide quiet and good lighting room
- Provide orientation clues in the environment, Like clocks, calendars, seasonal pictures, family photographs
- Provide newspapers to know the current events
- Use symbols to locate bathrooms rather than written signs
- Remove any environmental hazards
- Limit the number of family members, friends and visitors
- Provide frequent supervision.

4. *Promote communication and socialization*

As the patients will be disoriented confused and will have problems in understanding. The caregiver should:
- Approach to be very slow
- Introduce at each interaction and explain what for she is there.
- Verbal communication should be clear, concise and unhurried.
- Questions that require 'Yes' 'No' answers are best.
- Watch for emotional and nonemotional cues for evidence of perception of communication.
- Do not ask the patient to perform cognitive skills beyond his ability.

5. *Promoting independent functioning*

- Provide material for daily care available and accessible and encourage to do by themselves
- Routine must be made simple and consistent
- Enough time to be given to complete the task
- Reinforce the activity to gain confidence.

6. *Providing physical need of the patient*

Nutrition

- Provide food in small in quantity at frequent intervals
- Allow to eat at his own pace
- Provide roughage and green leafy vegetables
- Encourage fluids.

Sleep

- Control the patient's activity so, that he will stay awake during daytime
- Provide measures to facilitate sleep at nights.

Elimination

- Any problem of elimination to be assessed and cared

7. *Preserving family unit*: Care of a dementic patient is a full time and long-term care.
   - Patient's wife and relatives to be supported well
   - Education to family members regarding patient's condition and care to be explained
   - Family support groups and individual counseling may be organized
   - Linking them to some community based services may be tremendous help for the family

Nursing care of older adults can be effectively achieved through a special ingredient. The special ingredient in respect, the courtesy, consideration and esteem due each individual who has reached their age of life. This respect to be demonstrated in each nursing intervention.

ORGANIC AMNESTIC SYNDROME

Amnestic syndrome is characterized by a prominent disorder of recent memory and disturbance of time sense in the absence of generalized intellectual impairment.

Here there is no impairment of immediate memory. There will be severe impairment of recent memory or short-term memory (inability to learn new materials) to till in the memory gaps the parties uses imaginary events in the early stages of illness (confabulation) which disappears when the disease progress.

Causes of Amnestic Syndrome

1. *Thiamine deficiency*: The most common cause is chronic alcoholism. It is also called as Wernicke–Korsakoff syndrome. Wernicke encephalopathy is the acute phase of delirium proceeding amnestic syndrome when it becomes chronic phase it is called Korsakoffs syndrome.
2. Lesion in the posterior hypothalmus and hippocampal lesions of the brain due to:
   a. Vascular lesions
   b. Carbon monoxide poison
   c. Encephalitis
   d. Tumor in the third ventricle
   e. Surgical procedures.

Management

Management consists of:
- Treating underlying cause (treating thiamine deficiently)
- Supportive care for general conditions.

Other Psychiatric Syndromes due to Focal Brain Damage

This include miscellaneous mental disorder which occurs due to primary cerebral diseases, systemic disease or toxic substances.

Primary Cerebral Diseases

Epilepsy, limbic encephalitis, head trauma, cerebral neoplasm vascular cerebral diseases, etc.

Systemic Diseases

Extra-cranial neoplasm, endocrine diseases, metabolic disorder infection diseases.

Drugs

Steroids, levodopa, antimalarial, alcohol and psycho-active substances.

Management

- Basic investigations
- Finding out the underlying cause and treating.
- Providing supportive measures.

Nursing care consists of providing symptomatic and support care.

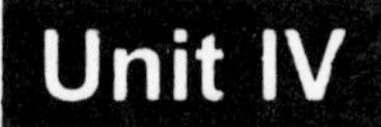

CHAPTER 21

Admission and Discharge Procedure

INTRODUCTION

Present day the admission and discharge in psychiatric hospitals made more simpler and the guideline is given below:

TYPES OF ADMISSION IN PSYCHIATRIC HOSPITALS

I. Admission as FVB (Free Voluntary Board)

Patient Brought by Family Members

Here the patient is brought to the hospital by a family member. After the careful examination if the; psychiatrist decides that the patient needs inpatient care, the patient can be admitted. Here the family member (spouse, father, mother, siblings), should give the consent for admission.

Patient himself/herself comes to the hospital

When the psychiatrist decides for inpatients care and patient is having insight patient can be admitted with his/her own consent. In both type income is assessed for the admission for payment in hospital.

II. Reception Order

a. It may be an under trial and found with behavioral problem. When the magistrate gives a letter to the psychiatric doctor asking to evaluate. If the psychiatrist finds that it is necessary to keep the patient in the hospital patient can be admitted to the hospital and inform the magistrate.

b. When a person finds any wandering mentally individual either a police or any public can bring the individual to the police station. Magistrate can give a reception order to a psychiatrist. If the psychiatrist decides to admit the patients', the patients can be admitted. If the patient can give the identify the relatives can be traced and get the consent for admission. If the family members are not traceable reception order is good enough to keep the patient in the hospital.

For both types of reception order admission, a periodic report to be submitted to the magistrate by the psychiatrist.

DISCHARGE PROCEDURES IN PSYCHIATRIC HOSPITAL

FVB (Free Voluntary Board)

If the patient is admitted with his own willingness the patient can be discharged when it is decided by the psychiatrist after due payments to the hospital.

If the patient is admitted after getting the consent of any family members at the time of discharges also the responsible family member to be informed and hand over the patient to him/her after the accounts settled if any.

DISCHARGE PROCEDURE FOR RECEPTION ORDER

If patient came with reception order the magistrate is informed periodically, the observations made on the patients by the treating consultant. This is sent by the medical superintendent of the psychiatric hospital. When the patient is considered to be discharged the treating doctor make a procedure call and do the de-certification measures. Then the patient can be shifted, from the inpatient care. This also should be signed by the medical superentendent.

Then the magistrate concerned is intimated and patient is shifted with necessary documents during the stay of patient in the hospital. The family members can be traced and they can take the patient. It can be done in case of wandering individuals. Individuals who are under trials should be handed over only to magistrate incharge.

Role of a Nurse During Admission

- The nurse working in psychiatric unit should have thorough knowledge of the rules and regulation of admission and discharge procedure given in Mental Health Act 1987.

  She also should know the institutional policies and procedures where she works regarding admission and discharge.
- Admission to the Hospital is an emotional trauma for the patient and his relatives. The nurse needs to be aware of the feelings of the parents or relatives and plan her approach and behavior accordingly.
- The nurse should look into the different written documents necessary to admission example, checking the income declaration, necessary deposit to

admission, getting signature in the consent form and other forms ensuring that patient relatives understands them completely.

- Vital sign and weight to be checked and recorded.
- Physical examination to be done importance to be given to findout any injury on the body and to be documented
- Mental status examination to be done (MSE) and written in the nurses notes
- Patients belongings to be checked and any harmful item like, knife blades, match boxes, etc to be removed from the patient to avoid accident or suicides in the ward.
- Any valuable things like wallets, cash, watches, jewellary, it should be removed from the disturbed patient and handed over to the relatives as there is strong possibility of loss or misappropriation. If no relatives are there the valuables to be safely kept as per the rules of the hospital and to be handed over at the time of discharge.
- Patient to be oriented to the ward, ward staffs.
- Rules and regulation of the ward. Timings of mealtime, visiting hours, etc. to be explained to patient and their relatives.

  Before assigning him a bed consideration to be given to his needs and of nursing staffs. It patient is suicidal or very psychotic he should be given a place where he can be observed all the time.
- Nurse should communicate to her collegues and other treating team, the necessary details of each admission and discharge which can prevent any legal issues.
- Nurse should show herself as a warm, caring and competent person, so that a more trusting and more therapeutic relationship develops.

Discharge

- When patient is to be discharged he should be encouraged to discuss about the issues and feelings towards discharge from the Hospital and living in the home environment.
- Instructions regarding taking medications regularly and its side effects should be informed to patient and his family member. Inspite of visible improvement the family is advised not to discontinue medication without medical advise.
- They should be told about the importance of regular follow up.
- The relatives should be educated about the early signs and symptom of relapse and report immediately to the doctor.
- The available community resources should be explored and continuity care to be arranged for the patient.

CHAPTER 22

Legal Aspects of Psychiatric Nursing

INTRODUCTION

The present day is the day of human rights. The nurse who deals with the general population, in general hospitals need to observe certain rules in order to keep her away from the hands of law. The case in psychiatric is so special where the legal and ethical consideration are to be taken care strictly to keep the nurses away from legal implications. In everyday psychiatric nurses are routinely involved in the complex life, events of their clients those may often involved legal issues. Not only they must make legal decisions for themselves, but they also must guide and support their clients when they face some legal issues in the life.

Psychiatric nurse, should take care of patient's rights, the legal role of nurse and the quality nursing care. These duties can be organized under the three roles of psychiatric nurse. Three roles care named as:
1. The nurse as a provider.
2. The nurse as an employee.
3. The nurse as a citizen.
Each of these roles has different responsibilities.

NURSE AS A PROVIDER

The psychiatric nurse has different role than a nurse who work in other branches of nursing.

Malpractice

The term malpractice and negligence often used inter changeably. Negligence has been defined as the failure to do something which a reasonably person, guided by those ordinary consideration, which ordinarily regulate human affairs, would go on doing something which a prudent and reasonable person would not do (Block 1974). The malpractice causing litigation against the nurses is the usual problem in psychiatric nursing. The professional negligence is called malpractice. It is defined as a failure of our rendering professional services to exercise that degree of skill and learning commonly applied under all the circumstances in the community by the average prudent respectable member of the profession with the result of those services on those entitled to reply upon them (Beis 1984), Most malpractice are filed under the law of negligent tort. The law is defined as "when a person or group must pay compensation for civil noncontractual wrongs caused to others". The malpractices can led to litigation against the nurses in psychiatric nursing.

Litigation

Law suits alleging malpractice in psychiatric diagnosis or treatment were rare few years, before. But now they appear growing in number the frequent complaints go to the court are:

1. Suicide of patient.
2. Improper medication.
3. Breach of confidentiality.

4. Injuries resulting from ECT.
5. Injuries resulting from restraint.
6. Homicides.
7. Sexual abuse.
8. Failure to obtain written consent for different procedures.

LEGAL RESPONSIBILITIES OF THE NURSE

Legal responsibilities include:
1. Reporting the patients details to coworkers.
2. Protect the patient from suicide and homicide.
3. Record the behavior in detail, it should be nonjudgmental.
4. Medication to be given carefully.
5. Keep the confidentiality.
6. Observe for any adverse effect of drugs.

Obtain written consent before any procedures, when a consent is taken there, are some criteria to be taken care of they are:
1. The person must be capable of consenting.
2. A person must have ability to refuse consent.
3. A person must have adequate information about the procedure.
4. The consent must not be illegal.

There are situation under which the treatment may be performed without obtaining informed consent. They are:

When a patient is mentally incompetent to make a decision and treatment is necessary to be performed without obtaining informed consent. These situations are:
1. When a patient is mentally incompetent to make a decision and treatment is necessary to preserve life or avoid serious harm.

2. When refusing treatment endangers the life or health of another individuals.
3. An emergency when the patient is on no condition to exercise judgment (Bais 1984, Gredstein et.al 1984).

Substituted Consent

If the individual has seen legally determined as mentally incompetent, consent can be obtained from the legal guardian if any. Substituted consent is that authorization given by another person on behalf of one who is need of a procedure on treatment, e.g. by guardian or patient's next kin. If no one is available the court can proceed to appoint a guardian.

Confidentiality

In nursing practice, it is an ethical duty to keep the information gathered about patient through interpersonal relationships and from indirect reliable sources. Stigma attached to mental illness is still prevailing. A breach of confidentiality of information about patients, their diagnosis, their symptoms, that behaviors and the outcomes of treatment can certainly affect the sort of their life in terms of employment, promotions, marriage, attainment, insurance, benefit, etc.

NURSE AS AN EMPLOYEE

This involves the practitioner's rights and responsibilities in relation to employer, colleagues and other team members. As employees nurses have the responsibility to supervise and evaluate those under their authority for better quality care for the patients. The nurse also should fulfill the responsibility of the employer towards patient care contract. The nurse also should appraise the employer the situation where the patient care is affected.

The nurse can claim certain rights also. The nurse can ask for the adequate facilities in working environment, adequate and qualified assistance whenever and wherever necessary.

NURSE AS A CITIZEN

The third role the nurse plays is that of a citizen. This role is particularly significant, all other roles, rights responsibilities and privileges are awarded to any individual because the individual is a citizen. Ours is a democratic government, which grants right to inherit, civil rights, property rights, right for any religion, right to protect from harm. The nurse as a employee and caretaker ought to consider her client also as citizens

PSYCHIATRY AND CRIMINAL RESPONSIBILITY

Criminal Responsibility

Section 84 of the Indian Penal Code of 1860 provides that nothing is an offence which is done by a person, who at the time of doing, it by reason of unsoundness of mind, was incapable of knowing the nature of the act or that what he was doing as wrong or contrary to law. The phase of insanity is generally brought forward during the trial stage. The accused is not found guilty, if insanity is unstabilized.

An amendment (1957) that includes irresistible impulses (covered under irresistible insanity) which are beyond the control of the lunatic is incorporated under section 84 of IPC.

At present four sets of criteria are used to determine the criminal responsibility of an offender who is mentally ill. The Mg Naughten Rule, The irresistible impulse test,

The Durham test or product rule and American Zan Institute Test.

Mg Naughten Rule

This is applicable in London. This law is originated in 1832 with the London trial of Damel the Naughten when he was tried for the murder of Edward Drummond, the private secretary of Sir Robert Peele Mr Naughten had suffered from delusions of persecution and had complained to public authorities many times. Receiving no help, however he decided to resolve the situation by himself. He began watching the house of sir Robert Peele and one evening, under the belief that he was shooting, Peele, he shot Edward Drummond. Mg Naughten was declared unsound by his attorney Mr Coclebarn and judge Teindal the Judge identified two rules from the (1) the first rule states that the individual at the time of the crime did not know the nature and quality of the act.

The second states that if he did not know what he was doing then he did not know that was wrong. Still this is used in courts of criminal law.

Irresistible Impulse Act

This is used along with Mr. Naughten's Rule. According to this the person may known the difference between right and wrong but finds himself impulsively drawn to commit the criminal act. It is usually necessary to show a lack of premeditation and that the urge was so strong that it would have been followed regardless of the circumstances. This test is defensive for sudden, violent behavior displayed under stress.

Durham Rule 1954

The accused person is not responsible of his unlawful act is the product of mental disease or mental defect.

In this the connection between the mental abnormality and the alleged crime should be established. This law was established in Columbia. The rule states that the accused is not criminally responsible if his act was the product of mental disease. That is why this rule is otherwise called 'product rule'.

Civil Responsibility

A person has no responsibility in the following condition if he proved to be a lunatic (Behaving abnormality).

Management of Property and Affairs of Insane

On the application of any relative of an alleged lunatic, the court may direct an inquiry to ascertain whether the person is of unsound mind and incapable of managing his property and affairs. There should be a medical certificate to show the degree of insanity which makes the individual unable to manage his property. In this matter the court can appoint somebody to manage the property. Under the transfer of property act (1987) only persons competent to make contracts are authorized to transfer this property.

Marriage—Under Hindu Marriage Act (1955)

A marriage between two parties either of whom was unsound mind at the time of the marriage is considered void. Divorce can be obtained on the ground of incurable unsoundness of mind for a specific continuous period. If lunacy starts after the marriage and continuous for two years even with treatment the other party can apply for legal separation and if the illness continue for more than three years, then the other party can apply for divorce. But the party has to pay the maintenance fee for the lunatic.

Testamentary Capacity

Indian Succession Act 1925 refers as testamentary capacity to the mental ability of a person to make a valid will. The requirement for a valid will are as follows:

a. A written and properly signed and witnessed instrument must exist. The testator must be major and free of force, undue influence or dishonest representation of facts applied by others at the time of signing the will. The testator is said to be of sound mind if he is capable of disposing of his property with understanding and reason. The tests used by doctor included test for orientation memory, concentration and the nature extent and value of his properties and the manner of his distribution. He should be asked in the absence of all attendance, together any pressure or influence has been brought on him by anyone.

b. Persons affected by an insane delusion can make a valid will if the delusion is not related in anyway to the disposal of property, persons can make valid will during lucid intervals. Partial drunkenness or the extreme of the age do not invalid the contract, if the reasoning power is intact.

Election or Right for Vote

No person with unsound mind can contest elections or exercise the brochure of voting. A person can be debarred from contesting election or exercising the vote by the court.

To conclude it is important for a nurse who practice psychiatric nursing to know the legal aspects concerned in this branch of medicine and nursing. It is in the interest of protecting herself and protecting her client from any legal problems. It is necessary for a better quality care in this field.

RIGHTS OF PSYCHIATRIC PATIENTS

1. Rights to communicate with people outside the hospitals through correspondence, telephone and personals visits.
2. Rights to keep clothing and personal effects with them in the hospital except for potentially dangerous objects.
3. Rights to religious freedom.
4. Rights to be employed if possible.
5. Rights to manage and dispose of property.
6. Right to execute wills.
7. Rights to enter into contractual relationship.
8. Rights to make purchases.
9. Rights to education.
10. Rights to habeas corpus.
11. Right to independent psychiatric examination.
12. Rights to civil service status.
13. Rights to retain licenses, privileges or permits established by law such as a driver's or professional license.
14. Rights to sue or be sued.
15. Rights to marry and divorce.
16. Rights not to be subject to unnecessary mechanical restraints.
17. Right to periodic review of status.
18. Rights to legal presentation.
19. Rights to privacy.
20. Rights to informed consent.
21. Rights to treatment.
22. Rights to refuse treatment.
23. Rights to treatment in the least restrictive setting.

CHAPTER 23

Indian Lunacy Act 1912 and Mental Health Act 1987

INTRODUCTION

In general hospital admission is a normal and easy procedure, where the individual came alone or with a relative seeking for medical help. When the condition needs impatient treatment the physician takes a decision and the individual agrees for the same. But in the psychiatric setup the situation is different. Many times the individual is unaware of his problem, so not willing for admission or he is aware but the stigmas attached to this condition may not allow him to agree for admission. But there are situations the psychiatrist has to admit the individual.

The individual

- May harm himself
- May harm others
- May deteriorate in physical condition which may lead to death.

To admit these individual though the individual does not agree there should be some legal procedure to protect the physician from the hands of law.

For this purpose every government, in India and abroad made Act in parliament.

Indian government made an Act in, 1912 which is known as 'Indian Lunacy Act 1912 and it is modified in

1987 as 'Mental Health Act'. If one examine these two Acts there are differences under different headings. Few major differences are given below.

Table 23.1: Difference between Lunacy Act and Mental Health Act

Topic	Indian Lunacy Act (1912)	Mental Health Act 1987
History	Derived from Mental Health Act of England and Wales (1959+1982)	It was a follow-up action of "Bore Committee".
Objective	To segregate the mentally ill patients from normal individuals as mentally ill may troublesome and dangerous to others.	a. To regulate admissions where no individuals are detained unnecessary. b. To protect the society from mentally ill individuals. c. To regulate responsibility for maintain changes of mentally ill persons admitted to psychiatric hospitals. d. To provide facilities for establishment guardianship or custody of mentally ill persons who are incapable of managing their own affairs. e. To regulate the powers of the government for establishing, licensing and controlling psychiatric hospital. f. To provide legal aid to mentally illpersons at state expenses in certain areas.

Contd...

Contd...

Incharge of asylums or hospital	Civil surgeons who do not have any knowledge about the case of mentally ill individuals.	Psychiatrist MD with license.
Preliminary information	*Asylum:* Means a mental hospital for lunatics established or licensed by central or state government.	*Psychiatric hospital or psychiatric nursing homes:* A hospital or nursing home established maintained by the government or any other person for the reference and care of mentally ill persons and includes a can convalescent home.
	Lunatic means an idiot or a person of unsound mind.	*Mentally ill person:* A person who is in need of treatment by reason of any mental disorder other than mental retardation.
Topic	*Medical practitioner:* Means a holder of qualification to practice medicine and surgery which can be registered in UK-1a in accordance with the law and includes any person declared by general or special order of a state government.	*Psychiatrist:* A medical practitioner possessing a postgraduate degree or diploma in psychiatry recognized by the Medical Council of India.

Contd...

Contd...

	Reception order: Means an order made by a magistrate or a police officer in a presidency town to retain under the provisions of this act a lunatic so found by inquiry. There was no renewal. Patient was there till death.	*Reception order:* Means an order made under the provision of this act, for the admission and detention of a mentally ill person in a psychiatric hospital or psychiatric nursing home made by the magistrate.
Board of visitor	Usually three, including inspector general of prison's appointed by the state government. 1. Medical officer 2. Inspector general of prisons. 3. Philanthropist or Mayor.	*Usually 5.* 1. Medical officer usually a psychiatrist. 2. Social workers –2 3. Director general of Health service-1 4. Inspector general of police -1
Working of board	Two or more of the visitors made regular visit to the asylum once in a month.	3 Of the board members visit hospital once a month. Review the admission_discharge of patients. Inspect the out patient and in patient suggest for improvement write the remarks and act as liaison between government and institution. The visitors will have no role in the admission and discharge of patient. They are not entitled to inspect the record of patients.

Contd...

Contd...

	Many visitors never attend the meeting and still continue as members of the visitors board.	If any members does not participate in three consecutive months, he cannot hold the membership
Admission on voluntary basis	*Ad on voluntary basis* *Major* application by a major to the medical superintendent with the consent of two members of board of visitors. *Minor* No provision.	*Ad - an voluntary basis* *Major* -Application by the major to the medical officer incharge of the hospital. No permission is required from the Board of Visitors. *Minor:* The nearest guardian can apply for admission on a prescribed form. *Admission under special circumstances* Any mentally ill patient who does not or is unable to express his/her willingness for admission as a voluntary patient. • The patient can be admitted and kept as an inpatient on an application made in his/her behalf by a relative or friend of the mentally ill person, if medical officer incharge is satisfied that it is necessary to do so in the interest of the mentally ill person.

Contd...

Contd...

		• But this patient cannot be admitted for a period exceeding 90 days or the reception order should be obtained. • The medical officer incharge of psychiatric hospitals or nursing home can keep a voluntary patient or a patient admitted under special circumstances for a longer period in the patient's interest provided the medical officer obtain a written consent by the patient's relatives.
Admission on Reception order	*Reception order on petition* *Admission through magistrate* The relative must have seen the patient personally for 14 days, supported by 2 medical certificates stating that the patient is lunatic and a proper person to be charge of and detained under care and treatment. One medical certificate should be by a registered medical practitioner and other should be by	*Admission under reception order* a) on application and a relative (husband wife, nearest guardian or friend) can apply to the Magistrate in writing supported by 2 medical certificates (one time Gazetted officer) for admission of mentally ill patient. No person who is a minor or has not seen the mentally ill patient within 14 days shall make an application. The medical incharge under whose care (hospital or nursing home) the mentally

Contd...

Contd...

a gazetted officer. Both must have examined the patient independently within 7 days of submitting the application.

ill patient is undergoing treatment under a temporary treatment order can give an application to the Magistrate that inpatient care is required for this individual for more than 6 months. b. On production before Magistrate the mentally ill patient (having violent behavior, dangerous to society detained by the police officer can be produced before the court within 24 hours. It should be accompanied by 2 medical certificates. Then the magistrate may issue a reception order. The relative who willfully neglect the patient may be punishable with a fine of Rs. 1000/-

Ad - in emergencies

If the mentally ill person is in danger and the medical officer incharge thinks so then such types of patients may be admitted. But within 72 hours the patient should be produced before magistrate or if he cannot be the magistrate is asked to come to the psychiatric hospital and get the patient examined and pass a reception order. Social

Contd...

Contd...

		worker of the hospital can go and make the order. These 72 hours are exclusive of the examination period. *Temporary treatment order* It is issued by the magistrate. It is done in such cases when there is a risk to the person's own life or to that of others. If the medical officer incharge feel that it is necessary to bring the legal authorities into picture, he can apply to the magistrate or the relatives can go to the magistrate to get an order issued for the treatment. This order is valid for 6 months
Reception order not on petition	*Admission through police* Any police officer incharge of a police station can assist any person whom he believes to be wandering lunatic or a dangerous lunatic. The arrested person to be produced before a magistrate who orders examination by a medical	*Power and duties of police officers in respect of certain mentally ill persons* Every police officer incharge of police station can take into protection/ custody any person wandering at large within the limits of his station and be produced before magistrate before 24 hours of taking him into custody and shall

Contd...

Contd...

officer. On receipt of the medical certificate of lunacy the magistrate issues a reception order for admission of the patient into the mental hospital. Police officers have been empowered to detain such patients for 24 hours, and then produce before magistrate. The magistrate can detain the patient for 24 hours, and then produce before magistrate. The Magistrate can detain the patient for 30 days, but not in continuity- that is to issue 3 reception orders of 10 days in each.

Reception order for criminal lunatic: A criminal lunatic is admitted on the order of the presiding officer of the court. The visitors of the mental hospital must visit the criminal lunatics at least once in 6 months.

not be detained beyond the said period without the authorities of the magistrate.

Admission of mentally ill prisoner: Reception order will be sufficient authority for admission. The reception order will cease to have effect on the expiry of 30 days from the date on which it was made.

Contd...

Contd...

Reception order after judicial inquisition Admission is important after inquisition. Any district court holding and inquisition regarding any person who is found to be mentally ill is of opinion that it is necessary so to do in the interest of such persons. By order this person can kept in mental Asylums and every order may be varied from time to time or evoked by the District court.	*Reception order after judicial inquisition* Same as that of Indian Lunacy Act, 1912. That, i.e. Patients 1. Who are psychiatric at the time of admission. 2. Person who had sound mind at the time of crime but develops psychiatric problem while in jail. 3. Sound mind when crime was committed and after punishment become psychiatric. 4. Psychiatrist can decide when the patient can be sent for enquiry.

Discharge procedures also are different in psychiatric hospitals/nursing homes. In general hospitals, usually the patient and the relatives will be eagerly waiting for discharge to get away from hospital atmosphere, hospital charges and routines. But in psychiatry many a time the relatives may be hesitating to take the patient home. The relatives are anxious about the further management of the patient. They may be apprehend to keep the patient at home along, to send the individual for work, etc. and there are occasions the relatives want to take these individuals for keeping them at home only to get their belongings or property making them legally unfit to manage them. So, every Government has taken care of these issues and made guidelines and in Indian Lunacy Act and Mental Health Act 1987, for the discharge of these individuals Guidelines are given below with the difference in both act.

Difference between Indian lunacy act and mental health act in discharge procedure

Indian Lunacy Act (1912)		Mental Health Act 1987	
Terminology	*Discharge procedure*	*Terminology*	*Discharge procedure*
Voluntary admission	The patient can ask for discharge by submitting an application in writing and the superintendent of the mental hospital has to discharge him within 24 hours of securing the application.	Admission on Voluntary Basis	The medical officer incharge of a psychiatric hospital or psychiatric nursing home, on her recommendation of 2 medical practitioner preferably psychiatrist, can direct the discharge of the patient.
		Admission on special circumstance	The relative or friend who gave application for the admission should give an undertaking that this individual who is mentally ill shall be prevented from causing injury to himself and to others.
Reception order on petition (Ad- through Magistrate)	The petitioner has to apply to the superinten-dent of the hospital who can discharge the patient if he is convinced that the patient is fit to be discharged.	Reception order on application or discharge of person or request	The applicant who feels that the patient has recovered from the illness makes an application for discharge to the Magistrate accompanied by a certificate from the Medical officer incharge of psychiatric hospital and if the magistrate feels that he is fit can order discharge of the patient.

Contd...

Contd...

Admission by the police	Patient can be discharged if the family members agrees in writing to take proper care of him and if the superintendent or the board of visitors are convinced that he is fit to be discharged.	Admission by police	Patient can be discharged if the family members agree in writing to take proper care of him. The magistrate is the responsible authority. The medical certificate is required by medical officer in-charge.
Admission of criminal lunatics	These patients who are fit to stand trial will have to be sent to the court. Those who are transferred from the prison will have to be handed over to the prison.	Admission of mentally ill prisoner	Same as of that of Act 1912
Judicial inquisition	Patient can be discharged only after another judicial inquisition.	Reception order on inquisition	After another inquisition and a copy duly certified by the district court stating that the patient is found to be of sound mind and capable of taking care of himself and managing his affair the medical officer than discharge the patient.

Contd...

Contd...

Review procedures for admitted patients	No provision	A patient in a mental health facility shall be informed as soon as possible after admission in a form and a language which the patient understand or all his or her rights in accordance with the present principles and under domestic law.
Supervision by central or state authorities	No provision	Supervision By mental health central authorities at the state and level
Supervision by central or state authorities Separate hospital for special categories	No provision	Scope for separate hospital for children for addicts, psychopaths, alcoholics, mentally retarded and the geriatric group.
Parole or leave or absence given to the patients to perform certain rituals or attend certain family function	*Parole* is an early form of release from the lunatic asylum and may be conditioned on the parole's receipt of the psychiatric treatment consistent failure to meet treatment appointments.	Leave of absence could be granted on application by the relatives (60 days) or other to the medical officer incharge and a signed bond is given stating that he or she can take proper care of the patient and prevent him from long injury to himself or others. Maximum period is 60 days.

Contd...

Contd...

	or comply with the treatment plan may result in legal sanction. During parole, person is in the role as a patient can leave the hospital, anytime and can be brought back forcefully, within a maximum period of 90 days.	
Judician inquisition regarding alleged possessing property and management of this property.	The court can appoint a manager to take care of the patient's property.	Provision for patient to have a guardian to take care of him and a manager to look after his property.
Escape and recapture	Should be brought back before 1 month otherwise has to be readmitted.	Can be brought back, no re-admission is required.
Shifting of the patient to another hospital.	No provision	The patient can be shifted from a hospital of one state to a hospital of another state with the consent of the government of that state.

Contd...

Contd...

Humanitarian provision	No provision as patient were under custodial care and were physical restrained.	No mentally ill person shall be subjected to any indignity, whether physical and mental or cruelty during treatment. No physical restraints can be used III. No letters or other communication sent by or to a mentally ill person under treatment shall be detained or destroyed.
Research	No provision	Research involving patients in mental hospitals is a human right issue. Clinical trials and experimental treatments shall never be carried out on any patient without informed consent.
Penalties and procedure for establishing a hospital or psychiatric nursing home	No provision	Any person establishing a psychiatric hospital or psychiatric nursing home requires a license otherwise he is punishable for a term of 6 months and a fine of Rs. 1000 or both.

Contd...

If both the acts are carefully examined Mental Health Act, 1987 has few advantages to be appreciated. They are:

- It is far ahead of similar acts of other countries
- It uses latest knowledge, in the field of mental health
- The public demands for better facilitates with flexible procedures are considered
- It attempts to concentrate on the psychiatrist's interest and well-being
- It has a humanitarian touch with keeping some of the right's of the individual patients.

NURSES RESPONSIBILITY

Nurses responsibility-While admitting and discharging the patient psychiatric inpatient units is discussed in detail in chapter-21.

The nurses should know the rules and regulations of both admission and discharge which is given in Mental Health Act, 1987.

- The nurse should know the institutional policies regarding the admission and discharge of psychiatric patient
- The nurses should be able to guide the patient and relatives about the Mental Health Act and institutional policies if needed
- The nurse should look into the different written documents necessary for admission
- The nurses should take signature wherever is necessary
- The nurse should document the necessary information while admitting and discharging these patients
- The nurse should communicate to her colleagues and other team members the necessary details of

each admission and discharge which can prevent any legal issues

- The nurse should see that the patient is prevented from any type of escape from the unit without necessary formalities
- If such thing happened she should inform the concerned authorities as early as possible with documentation.

As a whole the nurse should be equipped with thorough knowledge of admission and discharge procedures and also take the whole responsibility of keeping the patient in the unit till the discharge procedure is over and handover the patient to concerned person.

CHAPTER 24

Records and Reports

INTRODUCTION

Records and reports play a vital role in any organization whether it is an industry, hospital, even in private business, Government insists to have the record and record of any activity conducted in institutions for legal purposes. In hospital setup also it is not different.

DEFINITION

"Records are defined as a written formal legal documents of the patient's status, progress and treatment" (Goddard). It is also defined as a permanent account of events which can be reproduced on film or in writing.

PURPOSES

1. To collect information and to verify it.
2. To provide facts for services.
3. To serve as evidence to the care of the patient.
4. To provide basis for short and long-term plans.
5. To evaluate the care given and to offer teaching.
6. To prevent duplication of work.
7. To facilitate communication both horizontal and vertical.
8. To serve as guide for research work.

9. To judge the quality of work done.
10. To make out the progress and improvement.
11. To provide a means for determining achievements.

PRINCIPLES OF RECORDS KEEPING

1. Records should be with simple words, legibly written.
2. True facts should be utilized for legal documents.
3. Written for particular/specific purposes.
4. Provision for periodic review.
5. It is essential to have accuracy and completeness.
6. Provision for easy accessibility.
7. Adequate supply of stationary should be available.
8. Provision for confidentiality.
9. Records should be written immediately after review.
10. While closing, it should be signed by a responsible person.

TYPES OF RECORDS

Nursing Unit Records

Patient Records

i. These are necessary for good patient care.
ii. They help in teaching and research.

Medical Records

i. Medical orders should be written and put in its proper place in the patient's unit record.

Nurses Records

i. To furnish an accurate observation of the patient's condition.

ii. Record of the nursing care.

iii. Instructions to be carried out, should be entered.

Assignment Records

i. It is a record of nursing personnel and patient assigned to their care.

Time Record

i. It is a record which indicates the plan to obtain the care.

Census Record

i. Record maintained everyday from 12 'O'clock (MN) to next day 12 'O'clock MN.

Inventory Records

i. An itemized record of all articles under appropriate classification.

Narcotics Records

Nursing Office Records

Nursing Hours

i. Record rendered to all nursing personnel giving care to the patients.

Personnel Records

i. Record maintained for each one with all the particulars up-to-date.

Attendance Records

i. Record of attendance of personnel.

REPORTS

DEFINITION

It is defined as forms of communication prepared by individuals to pass information and understanding from one or more individual to another individual or group (Goddard).

PURPOSES OF REPORTS

1. Conveys factual information.
2. Amount of service rendered for specific period.
3. Helps in planning.
4. Evaluates the progress in patient care.
5. Helpful to communicate among professionals.
6. Interprets the services to public.
7. Helps in judging the quality and quantity or work done.
8. Helps in studying health condition.
9. Helps to provide better education services to students.

PRINCIPLES

1. Promptness is an essential factor for reports.
2. Communicate only the important information.
3. Avoid use of abbreviations.
4. Extranous material should not added.
5. Clear, concise, completeness should be maintained.
6. Proper expression and explanation should be given.
7. Telephone messages should be followed by written messages.

TYPES OF REPORTS

Nursing Unit Reports

Oral Reports

   i. Given by the nurse incharge on the condition and needs of the patients during handing and taking overtime.

Written Reports

   i. Written summary for the information about the condition of patient for several personnel's.

Taped Reports

   i. Helps to evaluate the quality of nurses' performances.
   ii. Provide information on new nursing problems.

Automated Intershift Nursing Reports

   i. Computerized nursing reports to resolve the problems in a comprehensive way by observation and caring of patient.

Nursing Office Reports

Monthly Reports

   i. A statistical report of information related to nursing department.

Annual Reports

   i.   Annual statistics for the covered items.
   ii. Recommendation for the improvement of services
   iii. Professional outstanding achievements, workshop, seminars, etc.
   iv. Provides an opportunity to point out the needs.

Varieties of Reports

    i.   Day, evening report and night reports.
    ii.   Inter-departmental reports.
    iii.   Inter-agency reports.
    iv.   Special report on unusual condition in the patient especially high-risk cases.
    v.   Reports on complaints.
    vi.   Evaluation report.
    vii.   Laboratory and other reports.

Hence Records and Report are Vital to the Profession

In psychiatric hospitals the nature and type of reports are little different. May include the mental status examination of the patients daily or twice for acutely ill-patients and alternate days for stabilizing patients and once a week for patients who are getting ready for discharge. It is done twice a month for chronically ill-patients.

Another tool used in psychiatric hospital is process recording. It is done everyday for patient who are admitted in psychiatric set up. The format for mental status examination and process recording are discussed in detail in different chapters of this book.

CHAPTER 25 

Psychiatric Emergencies

INTRODUCTION

Emergency is any sudden and unexpected situation which calls for immediate attention.

Psychiatric emergency is a disturbance of thoughts, feeling or actions for which immediate treatment is deemed necessary. These emergencies may cause threat to his existence (suicide) or threat to the people in the environment (homicide). So, immediate intervention is necessary to safeguard the life of patient, to bring down the anxiety of family members and enhance emotional security to others in the environment.

Psychiatric emergencies fall in two categories.
1. Emergency due to psychogenic causes.
2. Emergency due to organic causes

Whenever there is an emergency, it is necessary to obtain relevant information very quickly in order to differentiate between psychogenic and neurogenic causes. Be sure to find out past medical illness, hospitalization, recent accidents, serious illness, use of alcohol or drugs, history of fluctuation in consciousness and personal crisis, etc.

COMMON PSYCHOGENIC EMERGENCIES

1. Suicide or suicidal threat.
2. Violent behavior.
3. Excitement.
4. Panicky attacks.
5. Stuper or psychiatric patient.
6. Hysterical attacks.
7. Transient situational disturbances.

COMMON ORGANIC PSYCHIATRIC EMERGENCIES

1. Delirium tremors.
2. Epileptic seizure.
3. Drug withdrawal.
4. Acute drug induced extrapyramidal symptoms.
5. Drug toxicity.
6. Acquired immunodeficiency syndrome (AIDS).
7. Neuromalignant syndrome.

Suicide or Suicidal Threat

Suicide is a type of deliberate self-harm and is defined as a human act of self intentional and self-inflicted cessation (death).

In psychiatry a suicide and suicidal threat is considered to be one of the common psychiatric emergencies. If the patient is attempted suicide he is usually taken to a general hospital if he is threatening suicide he is usually brought to a psychiatric hospital.

Epidemiology

It is difficult to know the incidence of suicide and suicidal attempts in India because many cases are not reported due to legal problems and stigma. It is said one out of 12 attempts to commit suicide was found to end totally. The national suicide rate according to the police department is 8-9/ 1000 annually.

Common psychiatric illness where suicidal and homicidal behavior is observed are:
1. Major depression.
2. Schizophrenia.
3. Substance or alcohol abuse.
4. Hysteria.
5. Personality disorder.
6. Panic disorder.

Etiologic Factors Related to Suicide

Biologic Factors

- The neurotransmitter principally serotonin, dopamine, norepinephrine, etc. have been linked with emotional responses imbalance in serotonin plays a major role in regulating mood and influences occurrence of depression and suicide
- The role of genetic factors is also proved in association of suicide. A specific gene has been implicated in the redisposition to suicide
- Terminal or chronic illness also a factor for the causes of suicide.

Psychogenic Factors

- Self-directed aggression
- Unresolved interpersonal conflict
- Negativistic thinking pattern
- A reduction in positive reinforcement
- To end a feeling of hopelessness and helplessness
- Feeling of anger and hostility towards significant persons.

Sociologic Factors

- Feeling of isolation and aleniation from social groups
- Bio-psychosocial influences.

MYTHS ABOUT SUICIDE

- It is felt that suicide threat is just a bid for attention and should not be taken seriously
- Suicide/thoughts should not be discussed
- Only psychotic patient commit suicide
- Persons from good families will not commit suicide
- A failed suicide attempt should be treated as manipulative behavior.

FACTS ABOUT SUICIDE

- Any talk or idea about suicide to be taken very seriously and handled properly
- Patient should be encouraged to talk about suicide
- Suicide idea is cry for help. They want to live and wanting help from external sources to solve their problems. Allowing them to talk about their feeling, help them to relieve their tension and find new ways to solving their problem
- Not only psychotic patients even normal people suffering from psychological problems and problems with interpersonal relationship may commit suicide
- A failed suicidal attempt to be taken seriously as he may plan his future attempt still more carefully and well-planned.

RISK FACTORS FOR SUICIDE

1. *Age*: Males more than 40 ⎱ Indian context
   Females above 50 ⎰
   Age between 15-24 and ⎱ American context
   Older age 65 and later ⎰
   85 and above is most vulnerable.

2. *Sex*: Men have greater risk of completed suicide.
   Women have higher rate of attempted suicide.
   Male commit three times more than women.
3. *Marital Factors*: Being unmarried, divorced widowed
   or separated have high-risk.
4. *Physical and emotional symptoms*
   - Serious depression
   - Sleep disturbances
   - Extreme fatigue and loss of weight
   - Feeling of hopelessness/helplessness
   - Preoccupation with thoughts of death and dying.
   - Suicidal plan
   - History of previous attempts
   - Lack of social support and resources
   - Recent losses
   - Medical problems
   - Alcohol and other drug abuse
   - Lack of cognition and problem solving ability.

Five Levels of Suicidal Behavior

The following terms are used often in clinical setting to describe five levels of suicidal thought or action:
1. Suicidal ideation.
2. Suicidal threat.
3. Suicidal gestures.
4. Suicidal attempts.
5. Completed or successful suicide.

Management/Nursing Care

1. Take every suicidal threat seriously, however you suspect the seriousness of intention, since we can never be sure.
2. Round the clock vigilance of the patient is strongly recommended.

3. Spend some time with him talk to him allow him to ventilate his feelings, listen carefully.
4. Encourage the patient to talk about his/her suicide plans, methods, accordingly take necessary action.
5. Assure that you are there to support and any problem can be solved with discussion.
6. Provide safe environment for the patient.
    * Remove sharp objects, such as knives, scissors and mirror from the client's possession and access
    * Remove the toxic substances, such as drugs and alcohol and ensuring that unit medications are locked
    * Remove the clothing's, that could be used to self-destruction such as sarees, dupattas, neck ties, etc.
    * Do not allow patient to put bolts in the door and toilets. See that somebody accompanies him to the bathroom
    * Frequent check the toilet and bathroom, the patient might have planned to commit suicide.
7. Encourage the client to focus on strengths rather than weakness ones so that he becomes aware of his positive qualities and capabilities that have helped with coping in the past.
8. Explain the family members and relatives to take about that happy events of the family.
9. Sedatives may be given if suicidal ideas are very severe.
10. Have good vigilance especially during early morning hours.
11. Any clues of suicide, do not ignore. Research shows that 80 percent of people given clues before committing suicide.

12. Antidepressants ECT and psychotherapy may be given.

Violent Behavior

Violent or assertive behavior occurs in a variety of conditions like psychosis, personality disorders, epilepsy, alcohol and drug withdrawal, etc. It may be because of hallucinations and delusions.

Signs and Signals of Impending Attack

Before the patient may have violent attack he may have:
- Loud, angry speech
- Hyperactivity
- Intoxication
- Increased muscle tension
- Rigid posture
- Poor eye contact
- Increased autonomic system
  Diaphoresis of the palms or forehead red face, tachycardia, widened pupil, etc.
- Suspiciousness
- Verbal and physical threat
- Blocking the doors.

Management

1. Move very slowly, cautiously and deliberately do not startle the patient.
2. Talk with him in a calm, reassuring and natural tone of voice and ask him firmly what kind of help he requires. A scared or angry tone could cause the patient to become more frightened.
3. Calm, firm, and sympathetic approach is very necessary while dealing with these patients.

4. Try to make and keep eye contact with the patient. Looking in other directions may make the patient feel that he or she cannot trust the nurse.
5. Talk to him why he is doing so, and the consequences of his action.
6. Sometimes patient hence, may require some things like, food cigarettes, etc. provide if possible.
7. Putting the patient in cell (isolating the patient) helps to cool down many times.
8. If aggression is not reduced, he should be confronted by overwhelming free and should be sedated. Inj. Lorazepam 10 to 40 mg IV and Inj. Haloperidal 5 to 10 mg IV may be given.

Excitement

This is a severe form of aggressiveness. During this stage patient will be irrational uncooperate, delusional, paranoid assaultive, hallucinating and destructive.
It occurs in acute cases like:

- Schizophrenia
- Mania
- Confusional psychosis
- Alcoholic Intoxication
- Psychomotor or epileptic attacks
- Postictal phase of grandmal epilepsy.

Nursing Management

Take the help of 3 to 4 persons to catch the patient and put him down on the cot and give him injection Lorazepam and HPL IV. In severe cases of excitement, where threat to the life of others is anticipated. Blanket method can be used to catch the patient. That is one person must be talking with the patient continuously and one person should go from back with the blanket and cover his face and suddenly with the help of 3 to 4 persons. He should be caught and put down to give injections. This method is many times successful to give sedation to the excited patients.

- After the sedation the incident should not be discussed again with the patient as he may feel it as humiliation
- The injection may be repeated 4 to 6 hours or at shorter intervals to ensure that the patient remains underinfluence of the drug
- Then prompt treatment of the underlying psychiatric condition may be started.

Panic Attacks

Episodes of acute anxiety and panic can occur as a part of psychiatric illness or neurotic illness.

Patients during panic attacks will have:
- Palpitations
- Sweating
- Tremors
- Feeling of choking
- Chest pain
- Nausea, and abdominal distress
- Fear of dying
- Paraesthesia
- Chills or hot flushes.

Management

- Give reassurance, search for causes.
- Sedate the patient injection Diazepam 10 mg or Lorazepam Inj. may be given according to severity and continued with Tab. Lorazepam 2 mg twice or thrice a day till the symptoms are controlled.

Stuporose Psychotic Patient

Stupor is defined as a state of diminished consciousness in which the patient remains mute and still although the eyes remain open and may follow external objects.

The condition may occur due to organic or functional causes. The functional stupor may be due to schizophrenia, depression or hysteria. A careful history is very essential to distinguish among the three. The patient may be mute, motionless, may have echolatia, echopraxia and impulsive behavior.

Management and Nursing Care

- Care is similar to caring for a patient in coma
- Ensure patient airway
- Provide nutritional fluids for all the three kinds of stupor
- Check cardiac functions and stabilize it
- Draw blood for investigations before starting any treatment
- This should be followed by detailed work-up and treatment.

Hysterical Patient

A hysteric may mimic abnormality of any function which is under voluntary control. The common modes of presentation are:

1. Hysterical fit.
2. Hysterical ataxia.
3. Hysterical paraplegia.
4. Hysterical dyesthesia.

All presentations are marked by a dramatic quality and sadness of mood.

Hysterical fit must be distinguished from genuine fit.

All other hysterical presentation, which may be confirmed by:

1. Absence of physical signs.
2. Existence of psychological precipitate.

Management

1. Though the hysterical symptoms can create a panic among the relatives and others it is not serious concern.
2. Isolate the patient from the audience and relatives. Logical treatment is to make the patient realize the meaning of the symptoms and help her to face the stress and if possible remove the stressor. This will take a longtime.
3. Reassure that no harm would come to the patient and alleviate the anxiety of the relative and avoid secondary gain to the patient.
4. Abreaction therapy and psychotherapy may be given.

Transient Situational Disturbances

They are characterized by disturbed feelings and behavior occurring in the wake of overwhelming external stimuli.

Management

- Reassure the patient
- Allow the patient to verbalize and ventilate the feelings
- Mild sedation may be given
- Counseling by an understanding professional should be done

ORGANIC PSYCHIATRIC EMERGENCY

Delirium Tremors (DT)

Delirium tremors is the most severe alcohol withdrawal syndrome. It occurs usually with in 2 to 4 days of complete or significant abstinence from alcohol. This course is short. Death if occurs is due to cardiovascular collapse, infection, hyperthermia or self-inflicted injury.

Patient will have:

- Clouding of consciousness with disorientation to time place and person
- Poor attention span and distractibility
- Visual and auditory hallucination which are vivid and frightening
- Tactile hallucination of insects crawling over body
- Marked Autonomic disturbances with tachycardia fever, sweating, hypertension and papillary dilation
- Psychomotor agitation
- Dehydration with electrolyte imbalance.

Management

1. Keep the patient in a quiet and safe environment.
2. Give sedation usually Diazepam 10 mg or Lorazepam 4 mg IV given followed by Tab. DZM 10 mg Q6h to be given.
3. Plenty of fluids to be given.
4. Start IV fluids and maintain fluid and electrolyte balance.
5. Reassure patient and family.
6. Maintain body temperature, and vital condition .

Epileptic Furor

Following epileptic attack patient may behave in a strange autonomic way and become excited and violent.

Generalized seizures may occur in 10 percent of alcohol dependent patient usually 12 to 48 hours after heavy bout of drinking. Multiple seizures are more common than single seizures. Sometimes status epileptics may be precipitated.

Management

1. Sedation Inj. Diazepam 10 mg IV or Inj. Luminal 10 mg IV followed by oral anticonvulsant. Inj. Haloperidol 10 mg IV helps to reduce psychotic behavior.

Drug Withdrawal

Drug withdrawal is also a psychotic emergency. It will cause:

1. Psychological symptoms like, craving, irritability, excitement, agitation, confusion, disorientation hallucination, etc.
2. Physiological symptoms like diarrhea, vomiting, insomnia, rapid thready, pulse increased, lacrimiation, increased muscular twitching abdominal pain increased pulse, BP, etc.
   Common addictives drugs are barbiturates.
   Amphetamines, morphine and pethadine, opium and its derivatives hashish and marijuana LSD, etc.

Management

- Keep the patient in a quiet and safe environment.
- Give stat orders usually Inj. Diazepam 10 mg IV or Lorazepam 4 mg IV and sos.
- Tab. Donadin 1 mg 1-1-1 x 2 days
      Donadin   1-0-1 x 2 days
             0-0-1 x 2 days
- Calm approach is necessary. Avoid arguments and long explanation

- Provide plenty of fluids
- Provide finger foods which he can takes quickly
- Develop therapeutic IPR.

Acute Drug Induced Extrapyramidal Symptoms

Antipsychotics can cause a variety of movement related side effects collectively known as extrapyramidal symptoms (EPS). These are troublesome to clients and are major cause of noncompliance.

1. *Acute dystonia*: Muscular spasm that occurs in 10 percent of clients. This is often painful and frightening symptoms may be spasms of neck muscles (torticollis), upward deviation of eyeballs (occulogyric crisis) laryngospasms or opisthetonus.
2. *Akathesia*: Motor restlessness, pacing, rocking and foot tapping are common.
3. *Drug induced parkinsonism*: Mask face, drooling of saliva, tremors and rigidity.

Management

- Inj. Phenergan 50 mg IM stat to be given.
  This will relieve acute dystonias.
- For akathesia and parkinsonism Tab. Trihexypheridyl 2 mg tds is given.
- Explain the patient and families regarding the condition.

Drug Toxicity/Lithium Toxicity

Drug overdosage may be accidental or suicidal in either case make ask the attempt to find out the drug consumed.

- Take detailed history and examine the patient immediately
- Institute symptomatic treatment.

Common drug poisoning coming to hospital is Lithium toxicity. The symptoms are drowsiness, vomiting, abdominal pain, confusion, blurred vision, nystagmus, ataxia, stupor and coma, generalized convulsion oliguria and death, etc.

Management

- Stop medication
- Administer oxygen therapy
- Start IV lifeline
- Assess for cardiac arrhythmia
- Refer for hemodialysis
- Administer anticonvulsants.

Acquired Immunodeficiency Syndrome (AIDS)

AIDS related psychiatric emergency includes changes in behavior secondary to illness, along with organic symptoms, patient may have depression, anxiety, suicidal ideation and attempts, delusions, denial to the disease and treatment, reactive psychosis, hypochondriasis, mutism, agitation, restlessness, mania and withdrawal are associated psychiatric emergencies.

Management

1. Evaluation and management of suicide risks is the important task in emergency care.
2. Talk to the patient allow him to ventilate his/her feelings.
3. Good psychotherapy is essential.
4. Symptomatic treatment to be given.
5. Administer universal precautions.
6. Counsel the family members for crisis resolution.

Neuromalignant Syndrome (NMS)

Neuromalignant syndrome is a life-threatening complication that can occur anytime during the course of antipsychotic treatment.

Patient will have sudden hyperpyrexia (107°F) sweating, increased pulse, BP. The other motor behavior include muscular rigidity, dystonia akathesia, mutism and agitation. Lab findings indicates increased to creatinine, liver enzymes, plasma myolobin, etc. The symptoms usually evolve over 24 to 72 hours and untreated syndrome lasts for 10 to 14 days.

Management

The diagnosis is often missed in early stages as it will be mistaken as infection or increased psychosis. Men are more affected than women and young are more affected than older people. Mortality rate is 30 percent or even higher.

Treatment

It consists of:
- Discontinuing the drug
- Treating pyrexia
- Monitoring vital signs and electrolytes
- Starting IV fluids and maintaining fluid and electrolyte balance
- Maintaining intake and output chart
- Giving anti-Parkison's drugs and muscle relaxants.

When person recovers the drug treatment to be restarted. But low potency drug to be considered.

BIBLIOGRAPHY

1. Alphonsa Jacob. Handbook of psychiatric Nursing Vikas Publishing House Pvt. Ltd. 1996.
2. Bimla Kapon. A textbook of Psychiatric Nursing. Volume II, Kumar Publishing House, Delhi. 1998.
3. Fortinash, Holoday, Worret. Psychiatric mental health Nursing 2nd edition, Mosby company, 2000.
4. Frisch N & Frisch L. Psychiatric Mental Health Nursing. 2nd edition Delmar, Thompson learny, USA.
5. Kaplan H & Sadock B J. Comprehensive textbook of Psychiatry, Volume II, V edition William, Willkins.
6. M. S Bhatia. Aids to Psychiatry. 3rd edition, CBS Publishers and Distributors, New Delhi.
7. Seder, Lloyd and Rothschold. Acute care psychiatry, diagnosis and treatment Williams and Williams, A Waverly company, Philadelphia, 1977.

CHAPTER 26

Rehabilitation in Psychiatric Nursing

INTRODUCTION

Any episode of illness involves potential lasting changes in the individuals' level of functioning. The more serious the health problem, the greater is the possibility of a serious interference with the individuals ability to function productively in the community. Rehabilitation is the process, which helps the individual to return to his highest possible level of functioning.

Habilitation in Latin language means to 'live' Rehabilitation means to re-live or live again. It also means to restore, renovate to bring back to proper condition or to make it after illness.

DEFINITIONS

Rehabilitation is defined in number of ways as under:
1. Rehabilitation means restoration of the handicapped to the fullest, physical, mental, social, vocational and economic usefulness of which they are capable—(National Conference of Rehabilitation)
2. Rehabilitation is a bridge spanning the gap between uselessness and usefulness, between hopelessness and hopefulness, between despair and happiness.

3. Rehabilitation is an individual ability to function as efficiently and normally as his condition will permit following injury illness or accident. —(Blackwell, 1994).
4. It is an active process which seeks to reduce the effects of disease on daily life. —(Greenwood et al, 1993).
5. It is a combined and coordinate use of medical, social, educational and vocational measures for training or retraining the individual to the highest. Possible level of functioning ability. —(WHO, 1969).

In the field of psychiatry it is termed as psychosocial rehabilitation (PSR) Psychosocial rehabilitation is a process that facilitates the opportunity for individuals—who are impaired, disabled or handicapped by mental disorder—to reach their optimal level of independent functioning in the community.

It implies both improving individuals competencies and introducing environmental changes in order to create a life of the best quality possible for people with mental disorder who have impairment and disabilities.

It is perhaps relevant here to mention the WHO international classification of impairment, disabilities and handicaps (WHO, 1980). It says that condition can be looked at four levels.

1. *Pathology:* The intrinsic pathology and disorder.
2. *Impairment:* Loss or abnormality of psychological. Physiological or anatomical studies or function at organ level, the symptoms and sign.
   For example, loss of limb.
   Hallucinations, delusions, withdrawn behaviors
   This needs medical treatment
3. *Disability:* Lack of ability to perform an activity in a normal manner. The functional consequences.
   For example, Inability to write.

Poor self cares skills, social skills, occupational skills etc.

Treatment is training and retraining.

4. *Handicap:* The social disadvantage due to impairment and disability

   For example, Not getting job

   Treatment is Reservation and Assistance.

Psychosocial Rehabilitation Involves Series of Steps

1. Reducing symptomatology through appropriate pharmacotherapy, psychological treatment and psychosocial intervention.
2. Reducing introgency by diminishing and eliminating.
3. Improving social competence by enhancing individual social skills psychological coping and occupational functioning.
4. Reducing discrimination and stigma.
5. Getting family support.
6. Acquiring social support.

Rehabilitation As A Process has two Distinct Phases

1. *Treatment:* is the systematic way of dealing with illness
2. *Re-settlement:* is the re-establishment of a person in the community effectively. Here patient is helped to live independently with accommodation and employment despite of residual disability.

Rehabilitation starts from the time the patient becomes ill. A team approach is essential for rehabilitation, when the person become mentally ill various interventions are necessary to bring back the person to the previous level of working or living. Intervention by psychiatrist, psychologists, social worker occupational therapist, psychiatric nurse and other para-professional effort in essential along with family support.

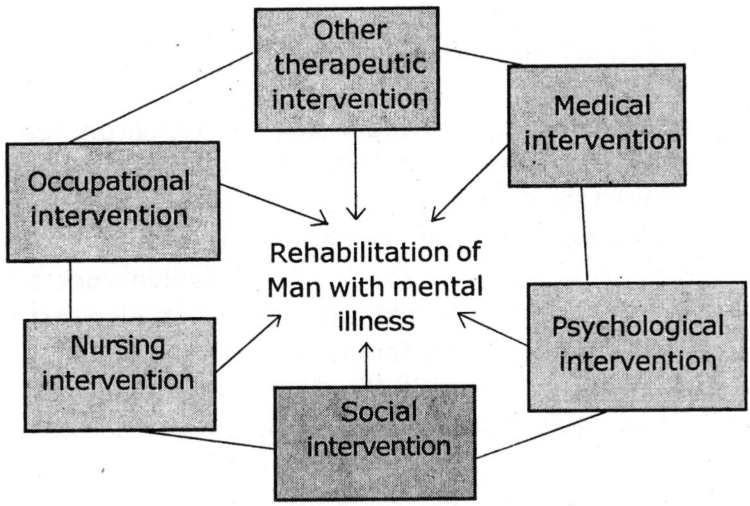

REHABILITATION IS THE EFFORT OF MULTIDISCIPLINARY TEAM

Principles of Psychiatric Rehabilitation

Anthony W Cohen M Cohen B identified some principles as basic to psychiatric rehabilitation settings they are:

1. The primary focus is on the improvement of the capabilities and competence of the person with psychiatric problems, even the most disabled. The alleviation of symptoms is secondary.
2. Insight is not a primary goal rather the focus is on the person's ability to function.
3. The provision of services is eclectic and uses a variety of therapeutic constructs.
4. Improvement of vocational outcome is a central focus.
5. Emphasis on positive expectations and hope is essential to the process.

6. A deliberate increase in dependency, as in sheltered settings, may be a first step in the process.
7. Active participation and involvement of the patient in rehabilitation.
8. Development of individual skills and environmental resources is fundamental in the rehabilitation process.

Rehabilitation aims at a comprehensive usually long-term approach to the management of psychiatric patients. This is an approach which involves not only the members of different discipline but also active participation of patient, family and community. It also continuously carries out the follow-up measures till patient is capable of living on his own with the existing social support.

METHODS OF REHABILITATION

In Patient Rehabilitation

a. Therapeutic Community

"It is a very special kind of milieu therapy in which the total social structure of the treatment unit is involved as a part of the helping process" (All social and interpersonal interactions are the therapeutic tools used to modify the patients behavior).

It was described as a new treatment in psychiatry by Maxwell Jones because it focused attention primarily on the psychiatric unit as a social system in which all members, staffs and patient, reciprocally influence one another for better or worse depending on the way in which the system functions.

The therapeutic community removes the patient from irritants of customary environments, theoretically giving him an opportunity of 24 hours a day to build a reward viable personality. All social and interpersonal interactions of the staffs are the therapeutic tools used to modify the patients behavior.

The important features are:

a. Communication.
b. Group meetings.
c. Interpersonal relationship.
d. Patient government.
e. Living and learning opportunities.

b. Habit Training

Habit training is another theoretical model based on the laws of exercise, frequency and recency. Long-stay patients especially mentally retarded, schizo-phrenic need this type of training, which involves re-education of patients, aims at establishment of good work habit, development of skills, manual dexterity, etc. It consists of:

a. *Living skills:* for example, personal hygiene, cooking, shopping, human relations self-control, money management.
b. *Learning skills:* for example, being quiet, maintaining punctuality, paying attention.
c. *Working skills:* for example, specific job tasks, job keeping, etc.

c. Social Skill Training

Consists of training the patient to acquire as many of his missing skills as possible to achieve re-entry in to the community. This includes teaching, living learning and working skill, e.g. personal hygiene, cooking cleaning, sewing, shopping, using recreational facilities communication skills, money management skills, etc. The training should be given one by one without making them anxious and by using various reinforcements.

d. Occupational Therapy

Occupation as a treatment facilities and provides for gratification of certain needs of the patients, both diversional and remedial types are being used for all the longstay patients. It helps to relieve anxiety and tension. Increased socialization and fulfills certain instinctual drives. Work is also ego strengthening for the patient, caters the need for action superiority, recognition and approval. It has a therapeutic effectiveness of its own.

Table 26.1: Potential skill activities needed to achieve goal of psychiatric rehabilitation

	Physical	*Emotional*	*Intellectual*
Living Skills	- Personal hygiene, Physical fitness, Using transport, Cooking, Shopping, Cleaning, Using recreational facility.	- Human relation - Self-control - Stigma reduction - Conversational skill	- Money management, - Use of community resources, - Goal setting.
Learning Skills	Being quite Paying attention, staying, seated, observing, being punctual.	Speech hearing, asking questions, following direction, listening.	Reading, Writing, Study skills, Typing.

Contd...

Contd...

Working skills	Punctuality, Specific job tasks, Use of job tools.	Job, decision making, Self-control. Job keeping, Specific job tools.	Job seeking, Job tasks. ...

e. *Recreational Therapy*

Includes activities which are more physical or game like in nature to develop contact of self with environment.

For example, Dance therapy, painting,

Music therapy, photography, etc.

It revitalizes the patient interest, and helps him to feel relaxed and refreshed. It is also an outlet for the expressions of emotions.

Community Rehabilitation

1. Partial hospitalization.
2. Half-way homes.
3. Foster homes.
4. Quarter way homes.

Partial Hospitalization

Obviously, it is not possible to admit all the patient, who are really now in need of the admission due to paucity of funds with a bed ratio of 1: 32500. It may be a far dream to be in a good position to cater for all the patients. So, the alternatives should also be thought of. One answer is partial hospitalization, which has to its own therapeutic effective apart from the cost effectiveness.

Partial hospitalization include:
a. Day hospitalization.
b. Night hospitalization.
c. Evening hospitalization.
d. Weekend hospitalization.

Day hospitalization: Day hospitalization is most popular and frequently used one in India and abroad. It has a structural treatment set-up, where the patient from homes and other institutions attends from 8 am to 5 pm. Evening they go to their homes.

It provides social, occupational and vocational, rehabilitation services. It also used to crisis intervention. The millieu has a therapeutic community orientation with an emphasis on small group formation and intervention.

The advantage of day hospitalization over in patient care:
1. There is no separation from family and friends.
2. They maintain their personal identity.
3. Most patient have lowered self esteem and total in patient care tends to lower the self esteem further and attaches a social stigma to the patient.
4. They have all professional contact in day time with various therapeutic activities and family contact in the night.
5. The possibility of regression, the face of life stresses is reduced
6. Day patient can maintain some social and vocational roles because they are at home in the evening and weekends.
7. The cost of a day hospitalization is less than that total hospitalization. The cost effectively of partial hospitalization compared to that of in patient hospitalization is 1:3.

Night hospitalization: This is another method of easing the transition from hospital to community life. Patient go to work in morning and return to the hospital at night. It will offer support until the patient feels secure enough for full discharge. This only for few weeks.

Evening and weekend hospitalization: This is a relatively newer alternative to the routine hospitalization. Indications for admission are not yet clear. However, one possible indication is when special therapeutic procedures like groups, etc. are contemplated for patients during the evening and weekends. In some countries for the relief of caretaker during weekends patient are admitted in this set-up.

Half-way Home

It is a transitional supervised residence assigned to help the patient after discharge from in patient settings. It is a temporary residence where various kinds of social skills training is given to this patients to make a readjustment to social life and employment in the community.

It attempts to maintain a climate of health and develop and strengthen normal capacities and normal responsibilities and prepares them for normal living in the community.

This is advocated especially for patient who might profit from group or dormitory living and can earn and help to pay their maintenance.

Foster Homes

Foster homes are another alternative, provided. They are secured to ensure that they do not give the institutionalized life but more like one in the family.

It is assumed that chronically ill-patient may live more normal life in foster homes than in mental hospital. But this is unsuitable to the aggressive and potentially violent, the suicidal, the sexuality deviant or alcoholic and other with nuisance characteristics.

Quarter-Way Home

It is a similar supervised residence where the patient lives in a facility in the hospital grounds. The facility is setup more like a hotel than a hospital and there is minimal nursing and attendant staff.

Acceptance of the Cured Patient by the Family

Rehabilitation process includes making the family members to accept the patient. Family support is very important to the successful rehabilitation of the mentally ill. So, it is necessary to:

1. Identify the problems of the family.
   For example, disrupted communications, mechanical routine life, unable to deal with the patients' problems and ignoring their own health.
2. Identify the family strength.
3. Encourage family to involve in patient care.
4. Provide psychoeducation.
5. Help them to help themselves.

Acceptance of the Cured Patient by the Community

This can be achieved through
- Giving health education to the community
- Working with local general practitioners
- Working with political system to develop community level policies
- Involving voluntary organizations
- Organizing group meetings in the community.

Re-employment

Patient should be prepared for re-employment:
- Provide a list of social agencies which can give appointment for the patient
- Invite representatives of various agencies to speak to patients group
- Escort patient to first agency contact.

Follow up to be Done to Evaluate the Success or Failure of the Individual Program and to know the Patient Functioning and Satisfaction

The success of program lies on patient involvement in occupation and decreased rehospitalization. As the patient becomes more independent in living, he requires less rehabilitation services.

ROLE OF PSYCHIATRIC NURSE IN, IN-PATIENT PSYCHIATRIC REHABILITATION

Nurses' role in rehabilitation consists of caring the patient with his/her social system. This requires the nurse should focus on three elements patient, family and community, i.e.

1. Develop good interpersonal relationship with the nursing care consists of patient.
2. Do the complete assessment of the patient
   - Socioeconomic condition of the patient
   - Abilities and assets
   - Disabilities
   - Type of work performed
   - Resources available in the family
   - And social support, etc.
3. Create a therapeutic environment in the hospital setup where patient can experience positive

relationship with others and motivated to learn and work.

4. Focus on fostering independence by maximizing the patients strength and potentials.
5. Provide an occupation as therapy which suits to his present condition and motivate him to do by giving positive reinforcement.
6. Assist him to become involved in social skill training program that uses cognitive and behavioral skills.
7. Find out the expectation of the family regarding the patient activity at home. In the same area train the patient to learn those activities.
8. Help the patient to involve in habit training program.
9. Encourage in participating social activities like games, sports, recreational programs, etc.
10. Provide necessary counseling and guidance sessions.
11. Teach the patient about relevant health care needs including physical health and mental health.
12. Act as the advocate in dealing with significant others in community for dealing any problem regarding the rehabilitation of this patient.
13. Assist the patient to develop a reliable social support system, identify and meet the family needs and help the family to accept the patient.
14. Provide psycho education to the patient and family about mental illness and coping skills to enable the patients successful living.
15. Refer the patient to a self-help group.
16. Assist the family to find out after care services in the community.

The psychiatric nurse should be the liaison between the other team members patient, family members and community to rehabilitate the psychiatric patients always.

BIBLIOGRAPHY

1. Kaplan et al. Comprehensive textbook of psychiatry III Vol Williams and Wilkins, Baltmore

2. Ekdaw and Alison. Psychiatric Rehabilitation A Practical Guide Champman and Hall 1990.

3. Stuart and Sundeep. Principles and practices of psychiatric Nursing 2nd edition The C.V. Mosby Company, 1983.

4. Principles and Techniques of rehabilitation Nursing 2nd edition C.V. Mosby Company 1961.

5. Stuart W Gail. Pocket guide series - Psychiatric nursing V edition Mosby Co 1998.

6. Kassler Henry H Lea and Febiger. The principles and practices of rehabilitation 1950.

CHAPTER 27

Pharmacotherapy— Nurses Role

NURSES RESPONSIBILITY DURING DRUG THERAPY IN PSYCHIATRY

Drug therapy has an important role in the management of psychiatric patients (of individuals with behavioral problems). Any other therapy is supported or supplemented by drugs therapy in psychiatry. The present form of drugs such as psychotropic drugs has a very short history. The role of neurotransmitters in normal and abnormal behaviors was not understood. Once the neurochemical therapy is established the drugs are being formulated in the management of individuals with behavioral problems. The research are still continuing to find out the exact pharmacokinetics of each group of drugs. In general, the psychotropic drugs are easily absorbed from gastrointestinal tract because most of them are lipophilic and are not highly consisted at physiological pH like many other drugs. They are absorbed faster in an empty stomach and in smaller amounts many of these drugs are metabolished in liver. And the metabolic end products are excreted through kidney. So, it is important to see the liver and kidney functions before starting these drugs as well as periodic evaluation of the same while patients are on these drugs.

The psychotropic drugs are distributed in the plasma where they bound to proteins. They easily pass from plasma to brain because they are lipophilic. For the same reason they enter fat stores from which they are released slowly. So, after the drug stopped also the patient can have the effect of drugs for a considerable period. The same way after the initial dosage taken, the action will start after a considerable time.

Measurement of Circulating Drug Concentration

The plasma concentration after standard doses of psychotropic drugs varies to substantially from one, to another. The expectation is the plasma level of drugs will help the clinician. But it is not. The relationship between plasma concentration and clinical effects are variable. The drugs are substantially bound to protein, the free fraction is more important which varies from person to person. The 3rd reason is the metabolites of some drugs are having therapeutic effect and others do not. The plasma levels also varies throughout the day, according to the time of drug intake.

Drug Interaction

When two psychotropic drugs are given together one may interfere with or enhance the actions of the other. Interference may be the area through alteration in absorption, binding, metabolism or excretion or interaction between psychodynamic effects.

Drug Withdrawal

Many psychotropic drugs do not achieve their full effect for several days, e.g. antidepressants may take two to three weeks to start acting. After the drugs have been stopped, there is often comparable delay before the effects are ceased or stopped.

Because of the special nature of these psychiatric drugs nurses who work with in psychiatric setup should have some special responsibilities in general.

They are:

1. The evaluation of all the systems should be done before starting the medications depends on age, illness, duration, etc. They include liver function test, kidney function test. Blood pressure, cardiac evaluation, etc.
2. Close observation is done to look for any extrapyramidal symptoms.
3. Observe and report any diarrhoea and vomiting especially when patient are on lithium.
4. Evaluation of vital signs is important.
5. Record of intake and output is necessary.
6. Salt intake should be increased when patient is on lithium.
7. Antacids are advised in case of any gastric irritation.
8. Blurred or impaired vision to be observed.
9. Complications like neuroliptic malignant syndromes to be observed and stop the medication immediately.
10. During mental status examination is necessary to see the adverse effect of the drug, e.g. antimanic can lead to depression or antidepressive can lead to mania.
11. Periodic drug level measurement is necessary for the drugs—Lithium, CBZ and Sodium valproates.

Classification of Drugs Used in Psychiatry

Psychotropic is a general term.

According to action of the drugs they are divided into the following categories.

1. Antipsychotic.
2. Antidepressant (Trycyclic, antidepressant, monoamine, oxydase inhibiters, etc.).
3. Mood Stabilizer.
4. Benzodiazepines-minor tranquilizers.
5. Anti-Parkinsons.
6. Psychostimulants.
7. Miscellaneous—Antiepileptics, enzyme intubator, Betablockers, etc.

The drug used in each category and their nursing implication are given in the following pages:

Antipsychotics

Antipsychotics are called major tranquilizers used to control the symptoms of psychosis such as hallucinations in bizarre or paranoid behavior. These drugs produce calming effect without significantly sedating the client.

The drugs are:

Typical Antipsychotics

- Haloperidol (Haldol)
- Chlorpromazine (Thorazine)
- Thoridazine (Mellaril)
- Fluphenazine (Prolixin)
- Trifluperazine (Stelazine)

A Typical Antipschotics = Serotinin–dopamine antagonists

- Clonazepam
- Risperidon (Risperdal)
- Olazapine (Zyprexia)
- Clozapine (Clozaril)
- Quietiapine (Seroquel)
- Ziprasidone (Zeldox)

They are associated with smaller risk of EPS.

Dose and Administration

Drug through injection produces significant clinical effect within 15 to 30 mts, whereas oral administration take 1 to 4 hours.

Side effects: Potentially troublesome side effect of antipsychotics include constipation, dry mouth, blurred vision, postural hypotension, urinary hesitancy or retension, weight gain and sedation.

Adverse effect: These effects are akathesia, dystonias tardive, dyskinesia and neuroliptic malignant syndrome.

1. *Akathisia:* Is a subjective sense of restlessness with a perceived need to pace or more continuously.
2. *Dystonia:* It is a sustained involuntary muscle spasms. Commonly involve the head and neck. One of the most dramatic dystonic reaction is oculogyric crisis in which extraocular muscle spasms forces the eyes into a fixed usually upward gaze.
3. *Parkinsonism:* This consists of tremor and an unsteady shuffling gait.
4. *Tardive dyskinesia:* This is a neurological disorder characterized by in voluntary movement most commonly of the tongue and lips. Grimacing, sucking movements, and lip smacking are among the most common tardive dyskinesia. It may be long-lasting despite withdrawal of antipsychotics.
   Tardive dyskinesia occurs in at least 5 percent of persons who have anti-psychotics for more than 1 year.
5. *Neuroliptic malignant syndrome:* This is a very serious complication of antipsychotic medication. Patient's will have sudden fever, rigidity, tachycardia hypertension and decreased levels of consciousness. Fever can rise to exceeding high levels and death

may occur. Treatment includes discontinuation of drug and administration of variety of medications like antiparkinsium, bromocriptive, dantrolene and benzodiazepines.

Most commonly used antipsychotic drug are given in table:

Table 27.1: Most commonly used antipsychotic drugs

Genetic name	Trade name	Mode of administration	Seda-tion	EPS	Dose range (mg)
Chlorpramazine	Thorazine	PO, IM,Po IV	3+	2+	100–1500 mg
Thioridizine	Mellaril	P O	3+	1+	100–800
Fluphenazine	Prolixin	P O	1+	3+	5–40 (1-5)
Trithioperazine	Stelazine	P O IM	1+	3+	2–40
Haloperidol	Haldol	P O IM	1+	3+	1–15 (2-100 mg)
Clozapine	Clozaril	P O	3+	1+	300–900
Olanzapine	Zyprexa	P O	3+	1+	5–10
Quetiapine	Seroquel	P O	3+	1+	300
Risperidone	Resperdal	P O	3+	1+	4–60
Clozapam					
Zipasidone					

NURSES RESPONSIBILITY

- Nurses should be aware of the side effects of the antipsychotic drugs and observe for the same in the patients
- If she observe early EPS symptoms, she should inform the doctor and Injection. Phenergan may be given in severe form. For mild EPS tab pacitane 2 mg may be given
- Maintain vital chart
- For female look for breast enlargement and maintain menstrual charting
- Weekly weight record should be maintained
- Watch for Neuromalignant syndrome which is a serious problem
- When patients are on atypical antipsychotics watch for agranulocytosis

- Any infections should be recognized and taken care in time
- Advise the patient to get up slowly from squatting lying down position
- Encourage the patient to have adequate food and fluids.

Antidepressants

Antidepressants are the drugs used to treat depression only given orally are typically well-absorbed and reach peak plasma concentrate in 2 to 6 hrs. Antidepressant effect is usually significantly delayed for at least 4 to 6 weeks after beginning the treatment.

There are three types of antidepressant.
1. Tricilic Antidepressant.
2. Monoamino oxidase inhibitors (MAOIs).
3. Selective serotonine reuptake inhibitors (SSRI).

TRICILIC ANTIDEPRESSANTS

The common tricilic antidepressants are:
1. Imipramine (Tofranil).
2. Desipramine (Norpramine).
3. Amitryptyline (Elavil).
4. Clomipramine.
5. Natriplyline (Pamelor).

Imipramine is more useful in depression of manic depressive illness. It is also useful in enuresis and anxiety attacks. Amitryptiline is useful when the depression is also associated with sleep disturbances. Desipramine is used when quicker effect is desired.

The side effects: of Tricilic antidepressants are:
- Dryness of mouth
- Palpitation
- Tachycardia
- Dizziness

- Postural hypotension
- Urinary obstruction and constipation.

Monoiamine Oxidase Inhibitors (MAOIs)

They are useful as second line of drugs for treating mood disorders but can only be used safely with careful monitoring in highly motivated clients.

- Hypertensive crisis is one of the dangerous effect. Hence if the patient has sudden severe headache BP has to be checked and taken care in time to avoid cerebrovascular accident.
- This drug has certain side effect when taken with foods that has pyramine.
- The foods to be avoided are cheese, curd and other foods which contain yeast, wine, beer, chicken liver, etc,
- Cough medication which contain dextromethorphan to be avoided.

Besides these the side effects of the drugs are:
- Hypotension,
- Dizziness,
- Vertigo,
- Fainling.

The common MAO drugs are:
- Phenelzine (Nardil)
- Tranylcypromine parnate

Selective Serotinin Reuptake Inhibitors (SSRI)

These are recently released. The SSRI offer excellent antidepressant effect with relatively few short and long-term side effects. They are used not only for depression and for other disorders like OCD migraine, chronic pain and alcohol dependency/abuse, etc. These drugs inhibit the reuptake of both serotonin and other neurotranmitters.

The commonly used drugs are:
- Fluoxetine (Prozac)
- Fluoxamine (Luvox)
- Paroxetine (Paxil)
- Sertraline (Zolofit)
- Citalopram (Celexa)

The common side effects are:
- Anxiety, headache, gastrointestinal disturbances
- Interference with sexual functioning
- Adverse effects are very rare but death have occurred following overdose of SSRI particularly when taken with alcohol.

Antidepressant Medications

Group	Drug	Chemical name	Dosage	Side effect
Tricylics and other	Amitriplyline	Elavil	25–300 mg	4+
	Doxepine	Sinequan	25–300 mg	3+
	Imipramine	Tofranil	25–300 mg	2+
	Desipramine	Norpramine	25–300 mg	1+
	Nortryptiline	Pamelor	30–100	2+
SSRI	Fluoxetine	Prazac	10–800	0
	Fluvoxamine	Luvox	50–300	0
	Sertraline	Zolofit	50–200	0
	Citalopram	Celexa	40	0
	Phenylzine	Nardil	45–900	0
MAOI	Tranylcypramine	Parnate	30–600	0

NURSES ROLE WHILE PATIENT IS ON ANTIDEPRESSANTS

- Encourage patient to take more oral fluids
- Observe for side effects of the drug and if any report immediately

- If the patient has sudden severe headache BP Should be checked for early recognition of hypertensive crisis and patient should be taken care to avoid cerebrovascular accidents
- Avoid taking alcohol
- Foods rich in pyramine to be avoided foods rich in pyramine are: cheese, curd, wine beer chicken, liver fish, sausage, alcoholic beverages
- Observe for suicidal ideas.

Mood Stabilizers

Mood stabilizers are used to control the symptoms of mania and once controlled to prevent recurrence. The most commonly used drugs are:
- Lithium (Lithobid)
- Carbomazepine
- Valporic acid: (Anticonvulsants but efficiently used to control the need)
- Divalproex

Lithium: It is most commonly used short-term long-term and prophylactic treatment for biplor disorders. It is also used as an adjunctive medication in the treatment of major depressive disorder, Schizoaffective disorders anorexia nervosa and in chronic aggression in both children and adults.

Lithium is neither a sedative nor a depressant and it appears not to affect mood in persons who do not have mania. Chemically, lithium is a metallic element closely related to sodium and is chemically recognized as sodium brain pathway. Typical dosage is 1800 mg given in three times per day. Serum lithium level to be maintained between 0.6 and 1.2 mEq/L levels above 1.5 mEq/L are associated with toxic effects. Very high levels may produced changes and potentially cardiac toxicity. So, lithium administration requires careful monitoring of serum levels.

Side Effects

Common side effect are: Thrist and polyuria
- Tremor, noticeable in fine motor activities such as writing, buttoning clothes, ètc.
- Chronic diarrhea.

Lithium toxicity depends on serum levels
- Signs and symptoms of lithium toxicity.

Mild to Moderate Intoxication (Lithium level-1.5.2 mgl/U)

- *Gastrointestinal*—vomiting, abdominal pain, dryness of mouth.
- *Neurological*—Ataxia, dizziness, slurred speech, nystagmus, lethargy/excitement, muscle weakness.

Moderate to Severe (Lithium level 2.0- 2.5 mEq/L)

- Gastrointestinal—Anorexia
  Persistent Nausea and vomiting
- Neurological—Blurred vision,
    Muscle fasciculation,
     Clonic limb movement,
      Convulsions,
      Delirium,
      Syncope,
      Stupor/coma,
      Circulatory failure.

Severe Lithium Toxicity

- Lithium level < 2.5 mEq/L—Generalized convulsion, oliguria and renal failure and death.

Management of Lithium Toxicity

1. Whenever the symptoms of lithium toxicity recognized. Immediately lithium should be discontinued. Patient should be instructed to ingest more fluids.
2. Physical examination should be done, including vital signs and neurological examination with complete formal mental status examination.
3. Blood should be sent for lithium level, electrolytes, renal function, etc.
4. IV fluids should be started and electrolytic balance should be maintained.
5. Serum lithium more than 4.0 mEq/l and with serious lithium toxicity hemodialysis is recommended.

Carbamazepine is most commonly used anticonvulsant but more widely used in management of mania. Peak levels may not reach until 24 hours after a dose. Divalproex resembles lithium in the absorption. Peak concentration reaches after 2-4 hours. Both carbamazepine and dival proex (valproic acid) have effects on brain electrical fuction. They reduce the brain susceptibility to disorganized electrical activity which may produce seizure disorder.

Carbamazepine is generally better tolerated than lithium but may seriously affect bone marrow functions and occasionally liver enzymes. Fatal agramulocytosis may result if blood counts are not carefully monitored.

NURSES RESPONSIBILITY WHEN PATIENTS ARE ON MOOD STABILIZING DRUGS

- The nurse should be familiar with the mood stabilizing drugs, indicates side effect and adverse effect.

- Liver function test to be monitored during treatment especially for carbamazepine and divalproex.
- TC (total count) and DC (differential count) to be done regularly.
- Nurse should teach the patient to be atleast for symptoms of loss of appetite, darkened urine, lightened stool, yellow color to skin profound fatigue that indicate impending liver failure.
- Patient should be observed for Steven-Johnson syndrome is a potentially total allergic skin condition. When patient's have skin rashes and such drug should be stopped.
- Careful monitoring of blood count to be done and any kind of infection to be notified early.

If the Patient's Were on Lithium

1. He should be observed for symptoms of lithium toxicity. Observe for gross tremors, ataxia, slurred speech, dehydration and altered consciousness and report.
2. Regular serum lithium level LFT (liver function test) and treatment (thyroid function test) to be monitered.
3. Monitor sodium intake.
4. Above 40 years ECG to be done regularly.
5. Stop the drug if fluid loss occurs and then restart.
6. Avoid pregnancy.
7. Activities which increases perspiration and inturn loss sodium should be avoided.

Benzodiazepines

Benzodiazepines are minor tranquilizers used in treating anxiety and insomnia and panic disorder. Nearly a dozen benzodiazepines are available for clinical use. The side effect are largely limited to sedation, interferes with safe driving and occasional amnesia.

The major adverse effects involve physical dependence withdrawal of the drug to be done slowly.

The commonly used drugs are:

Table 27.3: Commonly used drugs

Genetic name	Trade name	Clinical use	Dosage mg/
Alprazolam	Xanax	Antianxiety	0.75–4
Chlordiazepoxide	Librium	"	15–100
Clonazepam	Klonopin	"	1.5–20
Diazepam	Valium	"	5–20
Lorazepam	Ativan	"	2–4
Flurazepam	Dalmane	Hypnotic	15–30
Buspirone	Buspar	Antianxiety	10–60

NURSES ROLE

- Patient may be drowsy with these drugs. So, they should be avoided in work which causes harm to patients, for example, machinery work, driving, etc.
- Special precautions to be taken from patients.
  - Who abuse drugs.
  - Elderly persons who may fall.
  - People working in heights and dangerous work.
- Medicine should be tapered and slowly stopped.
- Observe for physical dependence.

Most Commonly Used Drugs

Most commonly used anti-Parkinson's drugs are given in Table 27.4.

Table 27.4: Most commonly used

Genetic name	Brand name	Tablet	Usual oral dose	IM or IV dose
Trihexyphenidyl	Pacitane	2 mg	2–5 mg/tds or bd	—
	Artane	2 mg		
	Trihexane	2 mg		
	Trihexy 5	per 5 ml		
Beniotroprine	Cogentin	0.5, 1, 2 mg	1-4 mg once or tds	1-2 mg
Procyclidine	Kemadrin	5 mg	2.5-5 mg tds	—

Anti-Parkinson Drugs

Anticholinergic drugs are primarily used as anti-Parkisions drugs for the treatment of medications induced movement disorder. Particularly neuroliptic induced Parkinsonim, neuroliptic—acute dystonia and medication induced postural tremors.

- The anticholinergic drugs are occasionally used as drugs of abuse because of their mild mood deviating properties.
- The most serious adverse effect is due to anticholinergic intoxication which is characterized by delirium, coma, agitation, severe hypertension and intraventricular tachycardia, hyperthemia and decreased bowel sounds.
- Treatment consists, discontinuation of drug and treated with physiostigmine (an inhibitor of choliresterolic) 1–2 mg IV every 2 min or IM every 30 to 60 minutes.

Psychostimulants

Psychostimulants are usually used with antidepressants for patient who are severely depressed. The stimulants are used in the management of narcolepsy, ADHD, etc.

The common drugs are:
- Pemoline (Cylert)
- Dextroamphetamine
- Methyl phenidate
- Cocaine
- Methamphetamine, etc

They are the major substance of abuse to be carefully monitored.

CHAPTER 28

Common Problems in Psychiatric Nursing and Interventions

Common Problems in Psychiatric Nursing and Intervention

Problems Identified	Nursing Diagnosis	Objectives	Nursing Intervention	Scientific Principle
Patient has very difficulty to establish trusting relationship. OR Patient not coming out of bed even with repeated persuasion. Not communicating even to simple question	Lack of trusting relationship. OR Patient has the fear of unknown, fear of unknown people, fear of surrounding due to psychopathology	To build trusting relationship	• Introduce yourself and your role in the unit. • Provide consistent environment. • Be honest in all interaction with patient. • Avoid topics and circumstances which the patient doesn't like. • Accept him as he is and give assurance that you are there to help him. • Keep promises and time of appointments.	Accepting as he is consistency, truthfulness and readiness to help will reduce the fear and starts the first step if good to establish the interpersonal relationship.

Contd...

Contd...

Common Problems in Psychiatric Nursing and Intervention

Problems Identified	Nursing Diagnosis	Objectives	Nursing Intervention	Scientific Principle
Not sitting in one place even for few minutes.	• Restlessness • Agitation • Increased anxiety.	To decrease the activity or to increase the concentration.	• Try to talk to him in his level of under-standing and interest. • Provide small activities in which he is interested. • Provide calm and non-stimulus environment • Encourage to do deep breathing exercises for few minutes.	• Talk and activities will increase the concentration and he decreases the excessive activities • Deep breathing exercises also increases the concentration and lessons the unwanted activities.
Patient is sitting alone not communicating and not even reacting to external stimuli.	Withdrawn behavior	To decrease the withdrawn behavior	• Spend time with the patient even if he is not reacting to your presence. • Convey your interest in caring him.	Environment stimulation can increase the different neuro-chemical substance which

Contd...

Contd...

Common Problems in Psychiatric Nursing and Intervention

Problems Identified	Nursing Diagnosis	Objectives	Nursing Intervention	Scientific Principle
			• Pay attention to non-verbal communication.	can stimulate the individual.
			• Direct the conversation at him expecting him to respond verbally but without demanding. For example, Calling him by name Looking at him, etc.	
			• Use simple short sentence and specific words	
			• Provide stimulating environment of light music and bringing him out where others are doing the activities.	
Patient is sitting alone and talking and laughing to self	Hallucinating	To decrease the hallucination	• Try to find out the content of the hallucination.	Idle mind increase the hallucination so work and
			• If the hallucination is of homicidal or suicidal take necessary care to protect him and others	activities will diverts his attention and decreases the

Contd...

Contd...

Common Problems in Psychiatric Nursing and Intervention

Problems Identified	Nursing Diagnosis	Objectives	Nursing Intervention	Scientific Principle
			• If possible find out the precipitating factors and avoid. • Do not agree with the hallucinate but do not argue because they are real to the patient. • Engage him in conversation. • Divert his attention in activities of his choice. • Allow the patient to ventilate his feelings of anxiety.	hallucination.
• Patient has false beliefs of Someone controlling him	Having delusions	To decrease delusions	• Develop trusting relationship. • Do not argue or agree with the delusions.	Divert the concentration where the individual have

Contd...

Contd...

Common Problems in Psychiatric Nursing and Intervention

Problems Identified	Nursing Diagnosis	Objectives	Nursing Intervention	Scientific Principle
• Someone perse-cuting him • Someone accusing him • Spouse not being faithful • People talking about him • Feeling of contamination, etc.			• Directly interject doubt regarding delusions as soon as the client seems ready to accept it. • Try to be with the patient allow him to ventilate his feelings and support his feelings. • Divert his attention by giving simple and interested activities. • If you know the content of delusion avoid the situations which can stimulate the ideas of delusions.	less time for delusional ideas.

Contd...

Contd...

Common Problems in Psychiatric Nursing and Intervention

Problems Identified	Nursing Diagnosis	Objectives	Nursing Intervention	Scientific Principle
Expressing to kill himself	Has suicidal ideas/attempt	To prevent suicide/attempt	• Spend time with the patient to find out about his feelings of suicidal and details. • Have close observation throughout day and night even when he goes to toilet. • Remove all the possible material and chemicals which can be used for committing suicide For example, Sharp instrument, ropes clothes, insecticide drug and razor. • Frequently talk to him and assess his mood and behavior. • Find out his interest in life it may be person or a plan to achieve	During depression patient will not be

Contd...

Contd...

Common Problems in Psychiatric Nursing and Intervention

Problems Identified	Nursing Diagnosis	Objectives	Nursing Intervention	Scientific Principle
			something in life on which he can keep his hope and avoid suicidal ideas. • Remind him of his assets and responsibilities for which he should live. • Keep him in a room/toilet where it cannot be bolted from inside.	able to identify his assets and responsibilities, ambition, etc. when they are reminded he may develop not to live.
Not able to sleep	Insomnia due to increased activity, hallucinations, delusions anxiety, depression, etc.	To promote rest and sleep.	• Decrease environ-mental stimuli • Provide comfortable bed and environment • Increase the activity during the day • Decrease nap during the day	• Calm environment can induce sleep activities in the day walk in the evening good food and hot bath can make

Contd...

Contd...

Common Problems in Psychiatric Nursing and Intervention

Problems Identified	Nursing Diagnosis	Objectives	Nursing Intervention	Scientific Principle
			• Use sedative only late night. • Give him good food in the night. • Give hot milk in night. • Encourage patient to walk in the evening and hot bath before going to bed. • Talk to him to make him to ventilate his feelings. • Find out the actual cause for sleep disturbances and try to avoid or treat accordingly.	the physically tired and induce sleep. • Avoiding nap in the day also helps to get sleep in the night. • Ventilating feelings can relieve tension and anxiety can relax the patient and promotes sleep.
Disturbances of appetite and regular eating	Increase Food intake to improve the nutritional status of the patient		• Find out the reasons for patient not taking proper food. • If it is due to less activities encourage the activities in the ward.	

Contd...

Contd...

Common Problems in Psychiatric Nursing and Intervention

Problems Identified	Nursing Diagnosis	Objectives	Nursing Intervention	Scientific Principle
	Suspicious of contamination or poison in the food	To lesson the suspicious on the food	• Provide tasty food according to the choice of the patient. • Serve the food attractive way. • Provide small frequent meals. • If the patient is catatonic tube feeding is advised. • Give finger foods to excited patients. • Give plenty of water. • Provide additional salt if patient is on lithium. • Find out details of the suspicious ideas. • Provide non-cooked foods like fruits, vegetables.	

Contd...

Contd...

Common Problems in Psychiatric Nursing and Intervention

Problems Identified	Nursing Diagnosis	Objectives	Nursing Intervention	Scientific Principle
			• Select and provide the food of his choice. • Allow the patient to be present while cooking the food. • Can allow the patient to cook the food himself. • Taste the food or eat the food along with the patient or before the patient eats. • Serve the food along with other patients. • Do not give medication along with the food. • Any color and extra flavor to be avoided.	• It lessons the suspicion as others also are eating. • It increases suspicion.

Contd...

Contd...

Common Problems in Psychiatric Nursing and Intervention

Problems Identified	Nursing Diagnosis	Objectives	Nursing Intervention	Scientific Principle
Patient is not having proper bowel movement or Patient is constipated due to psychomotor retardation/ or due to drugs.	Elimination deficit	To avoid constipation or to have normal stools.	• Asses the elimination • Increase fluid intake/ and include roughage in the food. • Provide active and passive exercises. • Remind the patient to go to the toilet on set time everyday. • Observe for any constipation and give laxatives if needed.	• Reduces constipation • This helps in better habits • Relieves constipation and helps to form regular habit.
Patient is not doing any productive activity in the ward	Lack of interest	To make the patient interested in activities and in life itself.	• Provide active exercises. • Encourage the patient to do ward activities For example Cleaning the ward making bed giving bath to other patient, etc.	Activity reduces the psychotic symptoms and help in increasing self-esteem.

Contd...

Contd...

Common Problems in Psychiatric Nursing and Intervention

Problems Identified	Nursing Diagnosis	Objectives	Nursing Intervention	Scientific Principle
Patient is not interested in his hygiene. • Not taking bath • Not brushing teeth • Wearing the same clothes everyday	Poor personal hygiene	To improve his personal hygiene	• Encourage to do his own work like washing his clothes, cleaning his bed, etc. • Provide work which is easy and able to achieve by the patient and satisfying to the patient. • Appreciate after completion of work. • Avoid competitive work. • Encourage the patient to do his personal hygiene with minimum help. • Provide clothing and toilet articles necessary and lead the patient to the action with positive suggestions.	

Contd...

Contd...

Common Problems in Psychiatric Nursing and Intervention

Problems Identified	Nursing Diagnosis	Objectives	Nursing Intervention	Scientific Principle
• Patient is very aggressive overactive/or hyperactive/ • Having hostile feelings towards other.	Aggression or hostility	To decrease aggressive feelings/ hostility	• Ensure that the patient attends to minimum care of brushing bathing, clothing, combing, etc. • When the patient had taken care of his hygiene express realistic appreciation. • Establish supportive nurse-patient relationship. • Make the patient to express his aggressive feelings in a quiet environment. • Teach him to practice the ways of expressing feelings without damage to either party.	Ventilation of feelings will decrease the intensity of the feelings. Patient learns the ways of expression of feelings even these are hostile

Contd...

Contd...

Common Problems in Psychiatric Nursing and Intervention

Problems Identified	Nursing Diagnosis	Objectives	Nursing Intervention	Scientific Principle
Patient is not socializing with other	Poor socialization	To improve socialization	• Encourage the patient to talk to others. • Introduce the patient to another patient who is quiet and coming out of depression. • As he improves, make him to join small groups later to a big group. • Observe for signs of anxiety if it is high take him out of the group. • Include him in other socializing activities of the group.	
Patient is not willing to take medications	Denial of sickness	To help the patient to accept and take medications regularly	• Find out the reason for not taking medicines. • Explain the need for treatment.	Patient refuses treatment because he enjoys the elated

Contd...

Contd...

Common Problems in Psychiatric Nursing and Intervention

Problems Identified	Nursing Diagnosis	Objectives	Nursing Intervention	Scientific Principle
			• Give drugs on time in correct dosage. • Observe the change in behavior due to treatment.	behavior or due to denial of sickness giving medication will reduce the above aspects and helps in improvement of behavior
Patient is threatening others, wants to assault or kill other	Homicidal ideas Homicidal threat	To protect the patient from injury to self and others	• Maintain calm, supportive environment in the room. • Do not keep sharp instruments near-by the patient. • Avoid arguments in the ward. • Have constant observation of patients behavior. • Avoid any kind of irritants in the ward which the patient doesn't like	Calm environment will help in reducing the excitement and irritation for the patient.

Contd...

Contd...

Common Problems in Psychiatric Nursing and Intervention

Problems Identified	Nursing Diagnosis	Objectives	Nursing Intervention	Scientific Principle
Patient is emotionally blackmailing the relatives/nurses/ others as he wanted drugs and other abuse materials.	Manipulative behavior	To reduce the manipulative behavior	• Understand the manipulative behavior. • Be present with the patient, ignore his symptoms but provide care. • Explain the relatives that patient is safe in the hospital with drugs/alcohol. • Encourage more fluids. • Explain the patient that these symptom due to withdrawal of drugs and are temporary.	Providing more fluids will help in preventing dehydration and promoting detoxification.
Patient feeling helplessness, hopelessness, and worthlessness.	Lack of self-esteem and self-respect	To improve self-esteem	• Encourage expression of feelings. • Nurses interaction and interest should make	

Contd...

Contd...

Common Problems in Psychiatric Nursing and Intervention

Problems Identified	Nursing Diagnosis	Objectives	Nursing Intervention	Scientific Principle
Patient is blaming himself for whatever is happening.			the patient to feel that he is useful. • Provide him a simple and easily achievable job and appreciate him after doing the job. For example, cleaning, bed making or paper bag making, etc.	
Patient is not having any diversion, looks blank.	Lack of diversional/ recreational activity	To increase patient participate in diversional and recreational activities	• Take the patient for walk. • Encourage exercises. • Involve the patient in small group activities. • provide the activities in which the patient is interested. • Put on music and allow patient to burn out their energy. • Switch on TV and allow them to watch.	

Contd...

Contd...

Common Problems in Psychiatric Nursing and Intervention

Problems Identified	Nursing Diagnosis	Objectives	Nursing Intervention	Scientific Principle
Patient does not do any religious activity.	Lack hope in God and religion, may be due to the feeling of hopelessness and worthlessness, and low self-esteem.	To increase patient participation in spiritual activities.	• Encourage the patient to come to the prayer room. • Arrange spiritual activities in the ward and encourage the patient to participate in the activities. • Encourage spiritual reading. • Encourage him to talk positively about himself.	Interaction with others in prayer room provide peace and calmness to mind and increase the hope in future life.
Patient to be discharged	Knowledge deficit	To provide knowledge about care after discharge.	• Advice the patient to take the medicine regularly and come for regular follow-up	Providing sufficient knowledge will decrease the

Contd...

Contd...

Common Problems in Psychiatric Nursing and Intervention

Problems Identified	Nursing Diagnosis	Objectives	Nursing Intervention	Scientific Principle
			• Teach the patient relatives how to identify the early signs of relapse and to come for treatment early. • Arrange for continuity of care in the community. • Advise him to get help when he is going through a crisis.	relapse rate.

CHAPTER 29

Community Psychiatric Nursing

INTRODUCTION TO COMMUNITY MENTAL HEALTH— NURSES ROLE

Community health care, through primary health centers in widely accepted and started functioning centuries back. Alma Ata declaration in 1978 by WHO has given a momentary to the concept. Every nation whether it is developed, developing or underdeveloped is fast aiming and reaching this global target of health for all, in its own capacity.

Community mental health nursing is the application of specialized knowledge to populations and communities to promote and maintain mental health and to rehabilitate target groups that continue to have residual effect of mental illness (Back + Routine).

Community mental health also taken due place in this effort. There are different reasons for the development and practice of community mental health, They can be listed as follows:

1. The number of cases are increased and the number of available bed and are not adequate.

2. The ratio of cases and professionals in this field is poor or inadequate.
3. Once the individual is admitted to inpatient setup the contact with the relations/family members become less and this can cause abnormal behavior.
4. The longstay in the hospital make the relatives feel the comfort of not having these individuals and they try to avoid to take back these individuals.
5. Advent of Neuroleptus can lesson the unmanageable symptoms of patient so that the management of these patients became easy in the community.
6. The etiological concept of behavioral disorders are changed and public is made to understand that this is a condition for which treatment is available and they can be kept in the community.
7. National Mental Health policy of different countries are written and started working to achieve its goals. One main objective of this policy is to involve family members in the treatment and rehabilitation of these individuals with behavioral deviation.
8. With all above said reasons many countries started closing down that large mental hospitals and many other decided and not to start any new hospitals or to increase the bed strength. These reasons directly caused the shift of focus of inpatient care to outpatient or community based care of mentally ill.

GOALS OF COMMUNITY MENTAL HEALTH ARISING

Goals should be inline with the general strategic community mental health of policies of each country. The main strategies are:
- Primary prevention
- Secondary prevention
- Tertiary prevention.

Primary Prevention

Aim of this is to prevent the occurrence of diseases. This is achieved through designing mental health—promotions, programs and health education packages. The programs are:

- Good antenatal care, perinatal and postnatal care
- Health education and on healthy parenting
- Health education on healthy family bondages
- Health education systems in the schools
- Healthy religious practices
- Giving awareness of expected problems in each stages of life and prepare with possible remedies
- Sex education in the schools and colleges to prepare for healthy marital and parental life
- Prepare the individuals in healthy aging and the acceptance of death as a natural experience in life.

Secondary Prevention

The meaning of this is once any disease on condition occurs handle them effectively either by individuals or by institutions to prevent the further complications. This can be achieved by:

- Anxiety and stress management programs individually or in classes dealing with rational fears.
- Resolving anger, resentment.
- Screening and identifying risk indications for self-destructive or self-abusive (suicidal) behavior and treatment.
- Give the awareness to the public to identify any early symptoms of abnormal behavior and report
- Give the information to the public the facilities and centers available for treatment if such condition.

- To put any of those program with action requires an advanced level of planning and education, therapeutic and management skills so it is practiced through the structural primary health centers by the community mental health nursing.

Tertiary Prevention

This stage of prevention plans to prevent the relapse of any condition which occurs once for this. Each professional should be competent in advanced skills and ablators to monitor the client. Again these professionals may not be able to supervise them individually. So, they conduct program individually or through mass media to make the public aware about the early symptoms of relapse.

To practice these strategies the community health nurses has different roles. The different roles are:

- As a consultant
- As a school nurse
- As a liason with other team members like doctors, politician, social workers, psychologists, etc.
- As crisis interviewer
- As a planner.

These services of mental health nurses is distributed mainly through:

1. Community mental health units.
2. Home visit.
3. Extension clinics.
4. Training the counterparts in other institutions in mental heath nursing.
5. Training the school teachers, politicians, NGO's ,village leaders different levels of preventions that in primary, secondary, and tertiary prevention.

THE PRINCIPLES OF COMMUNITY MENTAL HEALTH NURSING

The new kind has formulated five important principles for community mental health nurses. They are:
1. The search for recognized and unrecognized mental health needs.
2. The prevention of a disequalitarian in mental health.
3. The facilitation of mental health enhancing activities.
4. Therapeutic approaches to mental health care.
5. Influence on policies affecting mental health.

The Search for Recognized and Unrecognized Needs

- In order to practice this principle CMH nurses are required to research analyze and audit the mental health problems and its related causes
- The main concern for research can be in the field of reducing the rate of suicide and improve the functioning of people who are mentally ill

The Prevention of Disequalitarian in Mental Health

- This principle is practiced based on model of primary, secondary and tertiary prevention of Caplan (1961).

The Facilitation Of Mental Health Enhancing Activities

Long and Chanbers (1993) defined mental health as a process of equlirium both within and between the inner and outer self, the social environment, and the natural world in which people live in.

Every individual has self-awareness, self-acceptance and an ability to cope with changing life circumstances to balance the life, avoiding behavioral changes.

So, with the principle people can be made aware to empower to:

- Believe in themselves as unique individuals;
- Enable them to know themselves and others;
- Improve social relationships;
- Increase their understanding of life's meaning and purpose; and
- Realize their creative potential.

If the general population can practice these strategies they can make an equilibrium in themselves and keep away the abnormal behavior.

Therapeutic Approaches to Mental Health Care

The community has a tendency not to comply with treatment once the symptoms disappear. Here it is Community Mental Health nurses responsibility to give the awareness of the possibility of relapse of those conditions, because of the noncompliance. Here the nurse has to take care of care takers of these individuals. It may be family members, members of N.G.O's (non-governmental organization) or other professionals. This may be achieved by home visiting, visits to NGO's and other institutions where these individuals are cared.

Group interactions between patients and cares, patient alone, cares alone also can be arranged to promote the therapeutic approaches to mentally ill individual.

Influencing Policies Affecting Mental Health

Mental health goes close to the policies of each government. Policies has indirect influence on the mental health of population. The government also has direct influence by the people who has behavioral abnormality. The government has to plan to care these individuals which takes the national fund. Do CMH nurses have the responsibilities to help the government to solve its challenges.

The challenges are:

- Tackling the causes of inequalities
- Ensuring fast and easy access to therapeutic intervention
- Keeping patients fully informed all stages of their illness and recovery process
- Involving patients in their own care by working in partnership with them
- Designing action to improve both performances and the production of the fractional policies
- These challenges can be met by different strategies like
- Identifying the risk groups
- Establishing advocacy group and put them in action
- Executing self-help groups
- Arranging information centers.

To conclude a number of different models are advised and practiced in different parts of the word in community mental health nursing. But the fundamental principles of mental health for all is unchanged. So, it is important to note any health professionals working in any part of health care should plan and act in his own capacity to promote the mental health and maintain it. To greater extent any individual irrespective of his occupation is responsible to take active part in the promotion of health including mental health for this reason CMHN has to work to reach this message to every corner of the world.

COMMUNITY MENTAL HEALTH IN INDIA

In British era there were few mental hospitals and lunatic asylums to take care of individuals with mental illness.

Bed strength was not adequate to meet the demands of increasing incidence of mental illness. The availability of effective drugs, nonavailability of the indoor facilities for these individuals, along with the international influence. India also planned to start community development program in the field of mental health and illness.

Two centers were established in India for this purpose. In 1975 Chandigarh started a center, and in 1976 sakalwara in Bangalore also started a community mental health center.

The center at Chandigarh aimed to develop a model for rural psychiatric services. Later this project was supported by WHO with an intension of integrating mental health to general health services, and promotion of mental health care as a part of primary health care.

Second center was started in sakkalwara in Bangalore in 1976 as on part of NIMHANS. It aimed at conducting training program for doctors, multipurpose health workers to give basic knowledge about the detection and management of mental illness. It also has the program to make them able to detect and treat epilepsy. The staff of this center studied the needs of the rural population in one primary health care center. They also identified the mental illness in this given population. An integrated mental health care program along with the primary health care was given to 10,000 population around the center. (1980 to 1986).

In 1981, Director General of health services organized a national level workshop to consider a draft for mental health plan. This was held at All India Institute of Medical Sciences in New Delhi under the leadership of Professor N N Wig in July 1981. The draft suggested to initiate mental health services at center and periphery.

The above said draft was revised in 1982 by a small group of eminent psychiatrists. This body—the highest policy making body in the area of health recommended National Mental Health policy of India. This is known as NMHP of India's National Mental Health Program.

NMHP 1982

The magnitude of Mental Health problems is very large in India as in any part of the world. The number of professionals available for treating, them preventing the occurrence and promoting the mental health are very few. So with the help of W.H.O, the government of India conducted series of meeting to find some solutions. So a result to these meeting the government of India make proposals and recommendations, for better management of Mental Health problem in India. This programme is known as National Mental Health Program (1982) the objectives, approaches, salient recommendations are given below.

The objective of The National Mental Health Programme are as follows.

1. To ensure availability and accessibility of minimum mental health care fin the foreseeable future particularly to the most vulnerable and under-privileged or all Sections of population.
2. To encourage application of mental health knowledge in general health care and in social development.
3. To promote community participation in mental health service development and to stimulate efforts towards self-help in the community.

In order to achieve the above said objectives the programme has been designed to have the following approaches:

a. Integration of the mental health care service with the existing general health services:
b. To utilize the existing infrastructure of health services to deliver the minimum mental health care services.
c. To provide appropriate task oriented training to the existing health staff.
d. To link mental health services with the existing community development programme.

The programme will have three components, namely, treatment, rehabilitation and prevention of illness and promotion of positive mental health. The treatment programme has been planned keeping the primary health care approach as the sheet - anchor. At the same time, it consists of the creation of an appropriate referral system at various levels. It is proposed that the specialized psychiatric services should be made available at the district level. The other major responsibilities for the health personnel at the district level would be to provide training and supervision to the workers at the primary health center level. The mental hospitals, medical colleges, teaching institutions and mental institutes shall also be linked together into the national grid for the mental health care particularly in the field of education and research.

The rehabilitation sub-programme will develop services for the rehabilitation of the chronically disabled due to mental illness as well as mental retardation. This programme envisages linkages with the rehabilitation programme of other Ministries particularly the ministry of Labour and Social Welfare.

In the field of prevention and promotion, the sub-programme visualizes counseling services for common mental health problems like alcohol and drug abuse, delinquency and genetically inherited mental illness.

The salient recommendations are:

a. Mental health must form an integral part of the total health programme and as such be included in all national policies and programmes in the field of health, education and social welfare.

b. Considering the importance of mental health in the total development of society mental health aspects should be kept in view in the planning of activities for national development.

c. Appreciating the importance of mental health in the course curricular for various levels of health professional, suitable action should be taken with the appropriate authorities to strengthen the mental health educational component.

d. The practitioners of Indian systems of medicine should continue to play their respective distinct roles in the filed of health inclusive of mental health.

Recommendations of the Central Council of Health and Family Welfare Regarding NMHP

Recommendations made by the Central Council of Health and Family Welfare of Mental Health Programme in its meeting held on 18th to 20th August 1982 are as follows:

The Joint Conference considered the importance of mental health in the total development of society and appreciated that mental health is an integral part of total health and it should therefore be reviewed in that right. The Joint Conference recommends that:

1. Mental health must form an integral part of the total programme and as such should be included in all national policies and programmes in the field of Health, Education and Social Welfare.

2. Realizing the importance of mental health in the

course curriculae for various levels of health pro-fessionals, suitable action should be taken in consul-tation with the appropriate authorities of strengthen the Mental Health Education Components.

DISTRICT MENTAL HEALTH PROGRAM (DMHP)

This program started as a part of NMHP implementation. Initially 7 district started this program between 1997 to 1998. Gradually, other districts also started, reaching 25 district in 22 states of India.

Aims of DMHP

1. Training mental health team.
2. Increase the awareness of mental health and mental illness among the general public.
3. Provide service for early detection.
4. Provide data to center and state Governments for further planning.

   NIMHANS to be considered the Deemed Institute which carries out the activities to fulfill the central and state Government aims.

The Activities At CMH Unit Sakalwara

1. An inpatient facility with beds which opens for 24 hour of 365 days to meet the emergencies in general specially in mental health problems.
2. An out patient unit at Sakalwara which runs everyday except Sunday's and general holidays.
3. Weekly extension clinics—1 center.
4. Monthly satellite clinics in 5 centers.
5. Home visit everyday for detection, treatment, referral and follow-up of mental illness and epilepsy along with other general health problems.

6. Collects the data in different areas to help the center and state governments to do the future plan and budget.
7. Training and accentuation programs for different health professionals, doctor, nurses, social workers, psychologists, etc.

Mental Health Manpower Development

Manpower development was started in 1954 in All India Institute of Mental Health (present NIMHANS). In later other institutions also started different programs for this purpose. At present 75 percent of the available medical colleges conduct the specialize course for psychiatrist. Nurses, social workers and clinical psychologists also are given these degree in psychiatric speciality.

Involvement Of Families And Communities

Involving families and communities is a necessity of today. To have adequate member of trained people to look after the alarming number of mentally ill individuals is a dream for future. So, the training of family members and community is essential for this purpose different strategies are activated, activities are given as under:
1. Education programs during home visits though mass media, leaflets, etc.
2. Partnership with families and professional.
3. Self-help groups are formed.
4. School health programs are initiated.

The present day studies show the close relationship of neuroscience and psychiatry. So, all these programs, also has a indirect objective to detect, treat and prevent the neurological and neurosurgical condition.

Challenges in this field are quite time consuming and rewarding.

REFERENCES

1. David et al. Community Health Care— 2nd Edn Blackwell Science, 2001.
2. Community Mental Health Nursing Goldman Elaini—Appliton century efforts, 1972.
3. Oxford Textbook of psychiatry 2nd Edn, 1989.

Glossary

INTRODUCTION TO COMMON TERMINOLOGIES AND MEANINGS USED IN PSYCHIATRY—PSYCHIATRIC NURSING

This chapter deals with some terms and their meanings according to "FISH" abnormal psychology and Mosby's Medical Dictionary—1998, with some illustration by the authors themselves.

Acalculia: The inability to use the mathematical symbols is known as acalculia.

Affect: The outward expression of the immediate (cross-sectional) experience of emotion at a given time.

Agnosia Visual: The individual can see but cannot recognize what he has seen is called agnosia.

Agorophobia: The anxiety an individual experiences when he is away from home, or in crowds, or in a situation from which he cannot come out easily is called agoraphobia.

Aphasia: It is a term used to denote the inability to speak. But when a person can only understand, without responding, the term is called expressive aphasia. And when only the understanding is affected and expression is possible, the term is called receptive aphasia.

Ambivalence: Inability to decide for or against, due to coexistence of two opposing impulses for the same thing at the same time in the same person.

Anorexia nervosa: Refusal to maintain body weight for the age and height is called anorexia nervosa. It can also be expressed as a fear of becoming obese even when the individual is underweight.

Apathy: The absence or suppression of emotion, feeling, concern or passion, an indifference to things is called apathy. This condition is commonly seen in neurasthenic neurosis and schizophrenia.

Aphonia: A condition characterized by loss of ability to produce normal speech sounds because of the overuse of vocal cords, organic causes or psychogenic causes.

Aproxia: An impairment in the ability to perform purposeful acts or to manipulate objects. This condition is primarily neurogenic but occurs in severe forms.

Autism: A disorder characterized by extreme withdrawal and abnormal absorption in fantasy accompanied by delusion, hallucination, and inability to communicate verbally or to otherwise relate to people.

Infantile autism: A condition characterized by abnormal emotional, social and linguistic development in a child. It may be organic brain dysfunction. In which occurs before the age of three, or associated with childhood schizophrenia in later age.

Bestiality: Sexual intercourse of human beings with animals is called bestiality.

Cataplexy: An abnormal state characterized by a trance like level of consciousness and postural rigidity. It occurs in hypnosis and in certain organic and behavioral disorders like schizophrenia.

Circumstantiality: A speech pattern in which the individual in separating relevant from irrelevant information while describing an event .The individual may not only include every detail in a sequential order with the result the main thread of thought becomes lost as one association leads another. Very often the person needs to have questions repeated because the main point of answer, become lost in the confusion of unnecessary detail.

Confabulation: A fabrication of experience or situation recounted in a detailed and plausible way to fill in cover up gaps in memory. It can occur as a defence mechanism and is most commonly seen in alcoholics, head injuries and lead poisoning.

Delusion: A persistent adherent belief or perception held enviable by a person even through it is illogical, unique and probably wrong.
It is defined as An acute organic mental disorder characterized by confusion, disorientation, restlessness clouding of conscience, incoherence fear, anxiety, excitement and illusion see on page 326 of medication dictionary.

Dementia: A progressive, organic mental disorder characterized by chronic personality disintegration,, confusion disorientation, started detoriation of intellectual capacity and function affecting memory judgment and personality.

Depersonalization: Feeling of strangeness or unreality connecting oneself or the environment, often resulting from anxiety.

Depersonalization disorder: An emotional disorder characterized by depersonalization feeling in which a dreamlike atmosphere pervades the consciousness. The body may not feel like one's own. It is seen in different schizophrenia and in severe depression.

Dissociate amnesia (Dissociative Disorder): A type of hysteric neurosis in which emotional conflicts are so repressed that a separation or split in the personality resulting in an altered state of consciousness or a confusion in identity. Symptoms include amnesia somnambulism, fugue, multiple personality, etc. This disorder is due to the inability to cope with severe stress or conflict and usually occurs suddenly after a difficult situation.

Echolalia: It is also called echophrases—An automatic and meaningless and repetition of another's words or phrases especially seen in schizophrenia.

Echopraxia: Irritation or repetition of body movements of another person, a behavior exhibited by a schizophrenic individual.

Euphoria: A feeling or state of well-being or elation— An exaggerated or abnormal sense of physical and emotional well-being not based are reality or truth, disproportionate to its cause and inappropriate to the situation, commonly seen in manic or popular affective disorder.

Fetishism: Using inanimate objects or any part of the body not of a sexual nature for sexual gratification is called fetishism.

Homosexuality: Sexual activity and interest predominantly or exclusively towards individuals of same sex. Minority of male homosexuals exhibit pseudofeminine traits.

Illusion: A false interpretation of an external sensory stimulus usually visual or auditory.

Korsokoff's syndrome (Amnesia): A form of amnesia often seen in alcoholics ,characterized by a loss of short-term memory and an inability to learn new skills. It can be due to degenerative changes in the thalamus as a result of a deficiency of B complex vitamin, especially thiamine and B_{12}.

Masochism: Pleasure gratification derived from receiving physical, mental or emotional abuse. This may be from another person or oneself.

Mutism: An inability or refuse to speak. This may be due to a unconscious response to emotional conflict and confusion and most commonly observed in patients who are catatonic or depressed.

Neologism: A newly coined word or term. In psychiatry it is used to describe a word coined by a psychotic or delirious individual that meaningful to only that individual.

Obsession: A persistent thought or idea with which the mind is continuously and involuntarily preoccupied and which suggests an irrational act. The thought cannot be eliminated by logic or reason and usually causes a compulsive act.

Pedophelia: Sexual interest and activity of an adult is directed towards a child of the same sex or opposite sex is called pedophilia.

Panic : An acute, intense, overwhelming episode of anxiety, often associated with feelings of impending doom.

Sadism: An abnormal pleasure derived inflecting physical psychological pain or abuse on others is also called algolagnia. In psychiatry—a psychosocial disorder characterized by infliction of physical or psychological pain or humiliation on another person, either with a consenting or no consenting partner, to achieve sexual excitement or gratification. Usually, seen in men in severe cases it can lead rape and murder.

Schizophrenia: One of the large group of behavioral disorder characterized by gross distortion of reality, disturbances in language and communication, withdrawal from social interaction and disorganization and fragmentation of thought, perception and emotional reaction. It is divided into 5 major groups according to their predominant symptoms and the age of onset.

Stammering: A speech dysfunction characterized by spasmodic pauses, hesitations flattering utterness as mispronunciation or the transposition of letters within a word. Stuttering is synonymous.

Thought Broadcasting: A symptom of psychosis in which a patient believes that his/her thoughts are broadcasted beyond the head and others can hear those thoughts without he letting out.

Thought Insertion: A belief that a thought of other persons can be inserted into their minds without their knowledge and consent.

Tics: It is otherwise called mimic spasm. It is a steriotyped involuntary movement of small group of muscles of the face. This spasm is usually psychogenic and may be aggravated by stress or anxiety.

Transvestism: The pleasure derived from wearing the cloths of the opposite sex is called transvestism. Sometimes the pleasure is obviously sexual, but often it is used to relieve tension.

Waxy flexibility: Otherwise called cerea flexibilities. It is a cataleptic state, frequently observed in catatonic schizophrenia which the limbs retain in some position for an indefinite period of time. The position of the limb usually is abnormal and will be painful otherwise.

Word-salad: A jumble of words and phrases that lacks logical coherence and meaning often seen in schizophrenia.

Tardive dyskinesia: An abnormal condition characterized by involuntary repetitive movements of the muscle of face, the limbs, and the trunk. Commonly seen in Parkinson's and in individuals who use phenathiazen drugs for a long period.

Therapeutic community: It is a treatment facility in which the entire milieu is the part of treatment. The physical environment, the other client's, staff and the policies of the facility influence the prognosis of the individuals treated there. The concept is used in psychiatric setup as a integral part of treatment.

Token economy: A technique of re-enforcement used in behavioral therapy in the management of a group of people as in hospitals or in institutions. Here the individuals are rewarded for specific expected activities or behavior with tokens of appreciation in kind or words even with cash in later stages.

Trans-sexualism: When a person either believes that he or she is really of the opposite sex or just wants to be changed into the opposite sex, it is called trans-sexualism.

Zoophilia: An abnormal fondness of animals. A psychosexual disorder in the sexual excitement and gratification are derived from fondling of animals or act of engaging in sexual activity with animals.

Index

D

T